BESTSELLER

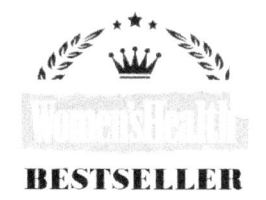

16:8 DIET
Intermittent Fasting For Women over 50

by Lisa Campbell

© Copyright 2020 by Lisa Campbell
All rights reserved.

This document is geared towards providing exact and reliable information in regards to the topic and issue covered. The publication is sold with the idea that the publisher is not required to render accounting, officially permitted, or otherwise, qualified services. If advice is necessary, legal or professional, a practiced individual in the profession should be ordered.

- From a Declaration of Principles which was accepted and approved equally by a Committee of the American Bar Association and a Committee of Publishers and Associations.

In no way is it legal to reproduce, duplicate, or transmit any part of this document in either electronic means or in printed format. Recording of this publication is strictly prohibited and any storage of this document is not allowed unless with written permission from the publisher. All rights reserved.

The information provided herein is stated to be truthful and consistent, in that any liability, in terms of inattention or otherwise, by any usage or abuse of any policies, processes, or directions contained within is the solitary and utter responsibility of the recipient reader. Under no circumstances will any legal responsibility or blame be held against the publisher for any reparation, damages, or monetary loss due to the information herein, either directly or indirectly.

Respective authors own all copyrights not held by the publisher.

The information herein is offered for informational purposes solely, and is universal as so. The presentation of the information is without contract or any type of guarantee assurance.

The trademarks that are used are without any consent, and the publication of the trademark is without permission or backing by the trademark owner. All trademarks and brands within this book are for clarifying purposes only and are the owned by the owners themselves, not affiliated with this document.

I wrote this book for all those women who have decided to change (for the better) their body, their health and their life by starting an exciting journey to discover new, healthy and wonderful habits ...

"What if I told you that everything you think you know about metabolism is a lie?"

You are about to discover the secret of 16: 8 DIET...

The simplest, quickest solution that almost nobody knows to lose weight definitively without regaining the lost kg...

CONTENTS

16:8 DIET 7
The surprising secret of a desperate housewife 7
Chapter 0 21
Before you start ... you have to set a goal! 21
Chapter 1 44
Let's start from the basics (Chronoalimentation) 44
Chapter 2 55
16: 8 DIET: The Secret Formula for Weight Loss 55
Chapter 3 65
Are you hungry ... or are you thirsty? Water: the secret of 16.8 DIET for weight loss in a healthy and fast way 65
Chapter 4 76
Green Tea, a Superdrink for burning fat 76
Chapter 5 84
Here's How To Gradually Eliminate Breakfast 84
Chapter 6 88
Find out how to further enhance the effects of this diet with the help of Ginger! 88
Chapter 7 99
Wellness Superfoods of the 16: 8 DIET for weight loss by eating 99
Chapter 8 128
70 yummy recipes 16: 8 KETO DIET burns fat 128
Conclusion 186

16:8 DIET
The surprising secret of a desperate housewife ...

My name is Lisa Campbell.

I'm 53. I am a housewife and mother of three children. I would like to tell you something personal about myself.

One day in September I succumbed to despondency and started to cry. I couldn't stop myself. I had hit rock bottom. I felt like a nervous breakdown was coming. It happened to me on a Monday morning just after I weighed myself in the bathroom. I have followed a strict diet for almost two months. I interrupted her over the weekend to give me a break and go back to living like a normal human being for a couple of days.

Now the scales showed that I was weighing 187,393 lb. I simply couldn't believe it! This meant that in one miserable weekend I had more than recovered every single pound I had lost in the past 3 weeks.

Maybe this doesn't sound like a big event, but it was a tragedy for me. I have tried to lose weight for the past 5 and a half years. I have tried liquid proteins. I have tried hypnosis. I tried to exercise. I had tried the sauna belts. For a period I even used dangerous dietary medicines. Everything about diets, I've tried it. The Zone Diet. Stillman's diet. The grape diet. The diet of the women's ski team. Etc. Etc.

You can quote what you want - I will have done it.

The results were always the same. I would end up trying hard and trying to lose a few pounds and then, on the first occasion when I would take a break, the weight would regularly go back. It had happened to me many times before, but this time it seemed like the last attempt. I didn't know who to turn to or what else to try. I was about to throw in the towel.

Do not get me wrong. I don't want this story to sound like tears. I am not telling you this because you feel sorry for me. There is no need in any case. My story has a very happy ending. It has a very happy ending because the next day I made a discovery that totally changed my life. I found an amazing way to lose weight that I never dreamed of could exist.

I won't tell you where I found this secret. However, I will tell you the following: I didn't get this information from a doctor. I didn't get it from a diet book. I didn't find it in a magazine. I didn't find it in a newspaper. I didn't get this information from any of the self-styled 'diet experts'.

To tell you the truth, I stumbled upon this information completely by accident while I was looking for something else. But all this does not matter. What matters is that he finally found an answer.

Let me tell you why I think my 16: 8 DIET secret is fantastic.

Dissolves fats quickly

First of all, this diet works quickly. It literally burns fat hour after hour. If you start it in the morning, you will continue losing weight before lunch. You will lose weight faster with this diet than if you tried to run 7 miles every day.

You will be able to measure the difference in your waistline within 24 or 36 hours. I think this is the fastest safe diet in the world. If you can find a diet that works even faster, I will buy it for you and I will gladly pay hard cash for it.

No hunger

I'll tell you a secret. You will never lose weight and be able to keep it on any diet without feeling hungry. It is an irresistible force. Sooner or later, willpower always gives way to hunger.

But this diet brings hunger to a definitive stop. You will never be hungry. For all intents and purposes, one of the unique characteristics of this diet makes it metabolically impossible for you to be hungry. For me, it means paradise.

76% more energy

This diet converts body fat into body fuel. From the fifth day of the diet your energy will ramp up. It will increase every day until the ninth day when it begins to settle. After that, your energy level will remain roughly the same. This new energy level is likely to be 76% higher than your current level.

****

"You will lose weight faster with this diet than if you tried to run for 7 miles every day. You will be able to measure the difference in your life within 24 or 36 hours. I think this is the diet fastest safe in the world. If you can find a diet that works even faster I will buy it for you and gladly pay hard cash to get it."

****

Simple and easy

This diet is very simple. It is easy to follow even if you eat continuously in restaurants. Don't count calories. You don't measure the portions. The only thing you keep monitoring is your weight loss.

Healthy and safe

This is not just a weight loss diet. It is also a healthy diet. It is safe. It is probably safer than the way you eat now. Don't play with your health. It's not worth it. Furthermore, it is not necessary.

You can lose weight fast with the 16: 8 DIET and also buy healthy every day you follow it.

WITHOUT exercise

You don't need to exercise to lose weight on this diet. Even if after the first few days you will have a lot of extra energy and you will probably become more active. But you will lose weight very quickly, whether you become more active or not.

Automatic weight loss

As soon as you go on this diet you will start losing weight automatically. You won't even have to think about it. Since you will not go hungry, you will probably forget that you are on a diet if it were not for the fact that you lose weight so quickly.

As you can say so far, I have found a rather brilliant solution.

I think 16: 8 DIET is the best way to lose weight I've heard of so far. You will lose weight quickly and you will never be hungry again. You won't have to count calories or measure portions. Your health will improve and your energy will increase. Cut off the moments when you weigh yourself, you will probably forget you are on a diet.

In short, this diet is quick, simple and safe.

There are three reasons why this diet works so well. These make it different from any other. Here are what they are:

Reason # 1

This diet has a different attack plan. It forces you to form new habits. These new habits are pleasant and fun. They make it possible to follow any diet throughout your life without ever feeling deprived. They make everything easier. It is so simple that you will wonder why you never thought of it yourself.

Reason # 2

This diet contains delicious foods that could prove to be absolutely new to you. I will ask you to eat at least one of these foods every day. These foods are what I call 'natural tranquilizing foods'. At the same time they will release new energy into your system, and will work to release any tension from your nerves and muscles, as well as to emotionally lift you. Trust me, it's hard to go on a diet if you're always angry and in a bad mood!

Reason # 3

This diet also contains another unique nutrient that releases the natural combustion power of your body system. This natural substance increases the number of calories your body burns every day, thereby allowing you to eat more without gaining weight.

A new dazzling body

This diet was a gift from God to me. I have a new body in great shape. I have lost 74,9572 lb. Now I am weighing 112,436 lb and I wear a size 38 (before I wore a 50). I have more energy now than I had when I was a teenager. I have better health than I can remember in the past. My friends say that I look younger than 15 years old. I have an inner peace never experienced before. I constantly feel good. Even better, my husband has fallen in love with me again.

Will this surprising little diet work for you?

I am sure yes.

All I ask is that you have enough open-mindedness to believe me even if I am only a housewife and not a doctor or something.

I wrote this book that tells about my secret diet: the 16: 8 DIET. It reads easily. It tells you exactly what to do step by step. And you can read it in one evening. Then, the next day you can start losing weight so fast that you don't believe your eyes.

Through this book I want to provide you with the tools that will help you, if followed step by step, to obtain concrete results and lose excess weight in critical points.

Reading these pages you will learn to organize your diet; you will educate your body to a varied and balanced diet, to a healthy lifestyle, you will learn to reduce stress (cause of abdominal swelling) and to raise the mood to obtain real and lasting results.

This program includes techniques and strategies to be applied daily to make sure you change your eating habits, eliminate excess fat and the waist problem once and for all.

With this book I want to help you get rid of all the ailments and discomforts caused by being overweight. Your physical shape, your appearance influence your mood, your way of acting and therefore every aspect of your life. As your appearance improves, your image and your self-esteem improve, and your self-esteem increases accordingly.

- ✓ *if you have weight problems and you can no longer hear yourself say that you just have to eat a little less and do some exercise;*

- ✓ if you are tired of dieticians, nutritionists, nutrition experts who don't listen and list you only and always everything you don't have to do and you don't have to eat;
- ✓ if you feel listless and apathetic;
- ✓ if you have tried many times to follow a diet without getting results;

If even one of the points listed is true for you, then this is the right book. Are you ready to start this program that will lead you to a healthy lifestyle and a leaner body, to feel fit and in place with yourself and consequently also with your neighbor.

If you are trying to dispose of excess weight, accumulated on the belly and hips, without getting results or with poor results; or if you lose weight but regain it immediately, then you must read this book immediately and put it into practice.

The reason that prompted me to write 16: 8 DIET is that I, like you and many people, have had weight problems for years and had to struggle with the discomforts caused by an out of shape physique.

I spent many years of my life in uncomfortable conditions due to my physical appearance. The strong overweight did not allow me to bring out the best part of me and did not give me the opportunity to enjoy life.

Very often these negative sensations, this strong discomfort, led me to eat what passed me, I was clouded by a nervous hunger and I did not spend time in the careful choice of food.

Food had become a "refuge" to cheer up my frustrations. Eating immediately made me feel better. I soon understood, however, that it was not the solution to my problem, quite the contrary!

The food increased my feeling of unease by making me feel even more awkward.

I also think about the luck I would have had and the time and money I would have saved if I had in my hands what you have available now: all the information and the solution to the problem of excess weight and unsightly belly in a only guide!

I worked very hard to find solutions, to find an effective system that would allow me to dispose of excess pounds and get the flat stomach I wanted.

I also wasted money buying alternative products, bars, diet pills and supplements. I wasted a lot of time and energy trying firsthand other methods and diets that turned out to be absolutely ineffective, in fact my body did not respond to any of these programs which made me angry, frustrated and intractable.

In addition, most diets are based on food restrictions. Diets focus on what cannot and should not be eaten instead of focusing on what is healthy, good and nutritious. With this program you will not have to focus on what you cannot or should not eat but you focus on what are "clean" and nutrient-rich foods, the healthiest foods that make you feel better, those to select for each meal or snacks.

I lost a lot of pounds and I found the pleasure of feeling fit and now I want to give you some tips, techniques and strategies that have been useful in reaching my goal and that I would have liked to have at the beginning of my adventure.

This book is the result of a long work of research, studies and personal experiences that you are now lucky enough to have all together and that you just have to put into practice.

By reading and practicing all the information and advice that I have the pleasure to give you, you can get rid of abdominal fat once and for all and regain your fitness and well-being.

You too, like me, can dispose of excess weight and get rid of it once and for all!

Don't delay, start today and remember that one step at a time you will reach the top of the mountain and the sooner you start the sooner you will reach your goal!

So what are you waiting for?

Immediately put into practice the secrets of the 16: 8 DIET and immediately get the sexy body you've always wanted!

"I'm sure you can do it too ...."

Enjoy the reading...

Here is what you will discover in this book:

Chapter 0
Before you start ... you have to set a goal!

Why set a goal? Because in this way you will drastically increase the chances of reaching what you want, of being able to get the body you want. And this is exactly what I want: that you can get much more than I dreamed of realizing the first time you opened this book.

Chapter 1
Let's start from the basics: chronoalimentation ...

Developed in recent years by an Italian doctor, Mauro Todisco (who by the way is one of the doctors who follow Dr. Di Bella), chrono-nutrition has proved to be the most effective trend for an optimal nutritional intake. But in this case it is not the usual bizarre diet, which every now and then is in fashion, but a real science based on precise hormonal cycles

Chapter 2
16.8 DIET. "The secret formula for weight loss"

Remember: One of the rules for being free is to question everything. If there is something that attracts you and you want to try, try it. If something sounds crazy to you, ask yourself why you think it sounds crazy, do your own research and experiment it before you have any prejudices and condemn it.

This is what I did with the 16: 8 DIET, I did a scientific research, I talked about it with a friend of mine, a dietician, I tried it first on me (with excellent results) then my friend a dietician extended the test on his patients, and the results were crazy, people were happy because they lost weight but without starving ...

Chapter 3
Are you hungry ... or are you thirsty? Water: the secret of 16: 8 DIET for weight loss in a healthy and fast way.

If you don't drink the right amount of water daily, your body cannot transform fat into energy and you struggle to lose weight even if you eat less. But how much water do you need to drink to lose weight quickly? You will find out in this chapter.

Chapter 4
Green Tea: a Superdrink for burning fat

This chapter will be dedicated to a Superdrink: green tea. Green tea effectively helps your body burn calories and fat by increasing your metabolic rate. Many studies show that including green tea in your diet (especially at breakfast) is of great help in promoting weight loss. But do you know which variety of you have to drink to increase your metabolism? You will find out here ...

Chapter 5
Breakfast: Here's how to gradually reschedule breakfast

In this chapter you will see that it will not be so difficult to get used to this new style of nutrition, after a few weeks you will be completely used to it and you will end up with a lean, toned and healthy physique!

Chapter 6
Ginger: Find out how to further enhance the effects of this diet with the help of Ginger!

Not everyone knows that ginger, also called ginger and known by most as a valuable food flavoring, is also a root with slimming powers:

• warms the body
• increases the temperature and perspiration
• helps eliminate excess fat and water

In this chapter you will find out how to use ginger by mixing it with other fat-burning herbs to cleanse the body, detoxify the liver, improve digestion, dissolve fats and quench hunger ...

Chapter 7
The Wellness Superfoods of the 16: 8 DIET for weight loss by eating

If you think you are alone, know that it is not so. The desire for food, for a certain type of food, is very difficult to combat, because certain foods stimulate the production of certain substances in the brain which, regardless of your will, create the desire to eat further.

Eating certain foods generates a food addiction which is the main cause of many health problems including being overweight and in severe cases obesity. I myself have experienced firsthand what it means to feel the unstoppable desire for food, so strong that it seems uncontrollable.

But there is a way out, there is a way to take control of the situation and no longer be addicted to food. In this chapter you will discover the way out ...

Chapter 8
70 yummy 16: 8 recipes KETO DIET fat burner

If you really want to push and increase your metabolism to burn more fat, then you should consider adding keto meals (especially at dinner) to the 16: 8 DIET.

Tons of celebrities are jumping on the 16: 8 Keto DIET bandwagon, and for good reason. The two systems work hand in hand to accelerate weight loss, not to mention many other health benefits. Fasting combined with keto meals is an extraordinary tool for improving your biology. It's free. It is universally accessible. It is adaptable.

Chapter 0
Before you start ... you have to set a goal!

"The secret to getting what you want is to know what you want"

Why do you have to set a goal?

Would you get on a bus without knowing which way it goes? In the same way we often find ourselves, for a variety of reasons, wanting something without having a direction, that's why it's important to set a well-formed goal.

Maybe you don't know, but only less than 5% of the population has a goal to achieve. Everyone says that setting a goal is important, yet almost nobody has one ... and what do you want to do?

Achieving a goal is very important to start building empowering beliefs for your new skinny identity. An important discovery I made while studying Neuro Linguistic Programming is that far better results are obtained when we turn our dreams into written goals, when we know where we are and where we want to go, it is simply a matter of finding out how to go from where we are where we would like to be and take the necessary steps.

For this reason, at the beginning of a project - such as the study of this diet for weight loss - it is worth taking some time to write down the reasons that lead you to read this book and the reasons why you want to lose weight. It is equally important that the goal is formulated in a particular way, because of the way our brain works. The goal must be "well formed".

A well-formed lens must contain what you want, not what you don't want. It must be specific and sense-based. You must be able to determine when you are going in the right direction. You need to know what it is that you can see, hear and feel when you reach your goal and are moving in the right direction. Management must be something you have control of and is in your power to do. Finally, the well-formed goal is something you have thought about properly, something worth pursuing. It must be good for you and have a positive impact in the different areas of your life, both in the immediate and long term.

So why set a goal? Because in this way you will drastically increase the chances of reaching what you want, of being able to get the body you want. And this is exactly what I want: that you can get much more than I dreamed of realizing the first time you opened this book.

Now, before moving on to formulating a well-formed goal, take 5 minutes and answer this question:

What is the goal and the result you want to achieve by reading this book?

Write down your reasons, the result you want to achieve and your goal in a notebook and then go ahead with the reading to understand how to formulate a well-formed goal.

How to formulate a well-formed goal

1) The first rule of a well-formed goal is that it be expressed in Positive to help the mind focus and visualize the result.

To the question: what is your goal, most people answer "I don't want to be fat anymore", "I don't want to wear size 50 anymore", "I don't want to eat chocolate anymore", "I don't want to binge anymore", etc. . The formulation of these statements focuses on what we don't want, rather than what we want. But formulating these sentences has an effect exactly opposite from what is our intention, because the brain does not recognize negation and therefore takes for good just what we want to avoid, everything that your mind vividly imagines, will lead you exactly in that direction. If you hope not to be wrong, in all probability it is what your mind will bring you to realize. Note what happens to our mind when we use the "non":

1. We give him a direction to go that is not the one he wants
2. We focus it on something we don't want
3. We value that negative image we have of the situation
4. We row against ourselves because we consciously decide where we would like to go and unconsciously go to the opposite

It would therefore be much more useful to formulate sentences that state what we want rather than what we don't want, so we will direct the mind in that direction.

-I want to be a slim and fit person
-I want to bring size 44
-I want to see myself beautiful without clothes
-I want to weigh 100 lb

Nobody knows their future and therefore you will never know in advance if you will succeed or fail in your goal, but for this you must help yourself with the internal language, using the right, positive words that will lead you towards the future that you imagine. So remove the word "don't ..." because, again, your mind does not recognize the orders given in a negative way.

I'll give you an example: if I tell you DO NOT think of a pink elephant, DO NOT think about it, DO NOT think of a pink elephant, ... what did you think of? To the pink elephant? I was sure ! Even if I tell you not to think about it, in that same instant your mind, in order to eliminate that image, must first represent it ... and you give a damn.

Remember that your mind does not recognize orders given in the form of negation. So if I say, "You don't have to be fat," what are you thinking about? Of being fat, of course. You can think of an image of yourself exactly as you no longer want to be. But how, your goal is another and keep in mind what you no longer want to be? As if to say: "today I watch a movie on TV that I don't like, would you see it? Surely not. You would certainly say "today I want to watch a movie I like".

So I repeat to you that the most important thing is that a goal is expressed positively. So you won't say, "I don't want to be fat anymore," you'll rather say, "I want to be thin." Now the first question you need to ask yourself to formulate a well-formed goal is:

What do I want, exactly?
What do I want instead of what I now have?
How do I want to be, instead of what I am now?
Remember to answer positively, I want ...

2) Your weight target must be specific and measurable to verify its progress and achievement with concrete data.

You say you want to be thin, I ask you, how much do you want to be thin? In fact, the goal you set yourself must be measurable, and in order for it to be, you must attribute a mathematical datum to it that allows you to understand exactly how close you are to your goal and when you reached it. It is a kind of finish line.

The desire to become skinny is not a goal, we have to talk about pounds and percentage of fat to reach. "Losing fat", "decreasing your waist", "toning", are not goals, but vague and poorly defined statements that at best we can fit between dreams and desires. But dreams and desires cannot be measured and evaluated in any way. There is no standard to measure progress and one day to say "yes, I have achieved my goal!". This is the main reason why many athletes, even genetically gifted, do not achieve excellent results. What incentive do they have to train harder, to follow a structured food plan for months and to refrain from counterproductive behaviors if a defined and structured goal is not present in their mind?

Goals are something very different from dreams. First of all they must be clear and measurable. There must be no interpretation of their achievement: a goal is centered or not, there is no middle ground. A goal must be as specific as possible, every time you define a goal, you must match the "thing" with a number: "weigh 14 lb less", "reach a percentage of body fat of 6%", "reduce the waist from 37 to 30 inches".

Defining the target numerically to make it measurable allows you to check and evaluate progress and understand if you have taken the right path or if you need to make corrections. A well-defined goal also generates self-motivation and induces discipline. If you know where you are at all times and you know where you need to go, you will always be motivated to give your best and do every day what is necessary to reach your goal.

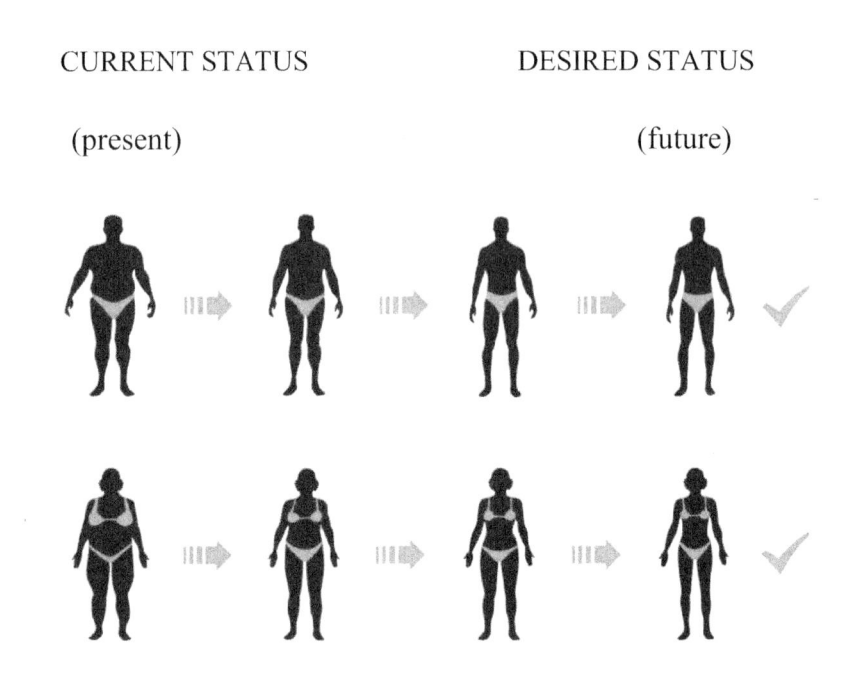

CURRENT STATUS   DESIRED STATUS

(present)   (future)

And remember that to be able to be every day as you want to become, there is no better motivation than seeing the tape measure tighten around your waist, the folds decrease and the weight on the scale go down! The path will not be easy: the more ambitious your goals, the more fraught with difficulties, there will be days when you will not want to continue, you will feel unmotivated, therefore you will have to be very determined. But to support you it will be enough to remind you that "now you are here and you have to get here".

A goal to be motivating must also be slightly difficult to achieve. Playing it safe does not help you, when you set a goal, you have to be a little afraid. The fear of not being able to reach it. This will generate that positive tension that will allow you to overcome your limits and improve. Be careful though. Defining a difficult goal does not mean that it must be impossible or unrealistic, setting a goal that is too ambitious or that is not within your sphere of influence will only lead to frustration. The goal must simply be challenging, if it isn't, you probably won't do your best to achieve it. Deciding to lose 44 pounds in 6 months is challenging. Losing 4 pounds in 6 months is easier and more realistic, but it does not represent an aspiration, in fact, after a few days you will already forget that goal.

"Aim for the stars to fall on top of the mountain"

Once you have set the main goal to be achieved, or the long-term goal, you will need to establish the so-called "intermediate steps", that is the reference points that you will need to understand if you are proceeding along the right path and in the correct time. For example, if the long-term goal is to lose 40 pounds, you will have to set short-term, monthly or weekly goals which, if on the one hand they will serve as reference points for evaluating your progress towards the final goal, from the other things will facilitate you from a psychological point of view in facing this path.

Focusing on losing weight at the rate of one pound a week is very different than focusing on losing 40 in six months. This allows you to keep yourself online and not say, when you reach the limit you had given yourself: "Ooops! I only lost 14 pounds instead of the 40 that I had thought, but a month is missing ... I won't be able to do it anymore! ". The sooner you know it, the better, so your course is more precise. It's a bit like having a compass, if you move a bit from the direction you had decided, it signals it to you in real time and you have the opportunity to correct the course. Measurability is very important because it imposes a time limit on your goal and distinguishes it from a dream. The deadline puts pressure on the completion of the job. Why do you think bills have a deadline to pay? Because otherwise nobody would pay them, for the objectives it is the same thing. A goal without a deadline, even if well defined, is not a goal, it is a chat from a bar or from social networks.

When defining a goal, you must always establish by when you want to achieve it. The time limits, in fact, as well as giving you the references to fix the intermediate steps, generate great motivation! To calculate the time it takes to reach your goals, you need to understand how much fat you can lose in a healthy way and minimize the loss of lean mass. The biggest mistake that most people who want to lose weight is that they don't take the time to lose weight properly. It is from this haste that almost all mistakes arise: eating too little, eliminating or excessively reducing carbohydrates, abusing proteins and too much aerobic activity, etc.

Your time goal should be to go as slowly as possible, lose as much fat as possible and not have any reductions in strength and energy during weight loss. To calculate how long it will take to reach your goals, you must therefore know how much fat you can consume in a healthy way and avoid the negative consequences we have talked about.

However if you don't want to calculate the fat mass and the percentages of weight to lose, know that the optimal amount of weight to lose, if you have to reduce the weight by 40/60 pounds, is a maximum of two pounds per week, if you need lose 10 to 30 pounds, the ideal is to lose one pound a week.

So if for example you weigh 200 pounds and you have 30% fat mass and you want to lose 40 kg (20% fat mass) your goal should be:

Positive: *I want to weigh ...*

Specific: *I want to weigh 160 pounds ...* (200 pounds minus 40 pounds to lose)

Measurable: *I want to weigh 160 pounds within 5 months ...* (half a pound a week for 20 weeks)

Before continuing with the reading, immediately write in your notebook, your positive, specific, measurable goal:

I want to weigh ...... pounds
by .... (write the precise date).

Done? OK let's go on ...

3) Your goal must be under your total responsibility so that you can achieve it without being dependent on others.

Achieving the goal depends on you, not on me, not on NLP, nor on the dietician. If you believe that buying this book gives you the motivation to lose weight just because you spent money, you are wrong, if you believe that going to the dietician and spending 300 dollars gives you the motivation to go on a diet, you are wrong. In this way you are unloading on me or on the dietician the responsibility that, instead, you should take on, that is to follow, with discipline, the book you are studying or the diet that you had from the dietician. So, if you do this, you won't make it, or this attempt will not last as long as all the previous ones.

I talk about it because I managed to get excellent results before you and because I too managed to follow the same procedure, and I still follow it, precisely because they are rules of life and not of therapy. I too have experienced them, I usually follow them and, therefore, I know the excuses that everyone invents to escape from them.

So the achievement of your goal must not depend on this book, but it will be the means to achieve the goal, then you will be committed to following exactly the strategies that I will give you in the book, only if you follow what you read literally, and you will put into practice what I will say to do, then, you will be able to say that you have or have not reached the goal because of the book or because of you. You have to commit yourself. The word "commitment" means "to dedicate oneself unconditionally and responsibly", that is to give 100% of all that is available to achieve the goal of losing weight. I am giving you a very powerful tool to help you lose weight, but the responsibility of using it well depends only on you ...

So your goal will be:

I want to weigh ...... pounds
by .... (write the precise date),
and I really strive to achieve this!

Write it in your notebook ...

4) Your goal must maintain the advantages of the present, so that there are no internal self-sabotages.

Now ask yourself what advantages you have in not losing weight, in remaining as you are now. Maybe you have a little belly or you have the classic "donut", but you are doing well, so much your husband likes a little "flesh". At least so you stay calm, you don't have to play sports, you don't have to try hard, you don't have to commit yourself, you don't have to take responsibility, you can eat whatever you want. Maybe eating a dessert makes you relax. It's a bit like having the habit of smoking. We would like to quit but we cannot, because there are too many secondary advantages that our current habits guarantee us. The secondary benefits are unconscious benefits that an addiction, like smoking a cigarette, offers us: those who smoke usually do it to relax, so if they stop, they don't know how else to relax. "

We can take another example with depressed people who take pleasure in the fact that in times of crisis, their family members rush, giving them attention and affection. Depressed people associate the crisis with the love of loved ones and, therefore, unconsciously, their malaise becomes a kind of drug they cannot do without. With this example I want to make you understand that the idea of not being able to do without secondary benefits is capable of profoundly conditioning a person's psyche, limiting it in achieving its goal. So, in setting the goal and in pursuing it, you must also make sure that you can somehow preserve the advantages of the present.

If eating continuously makes you relax or stress relieves you, know that you can also relax in other ways, for example with a hobby, with a nice hot bath, listening to music, reading a book, in short, relaxing without damaging your line, just as you can relieve stress by doing sports, walking or having sex (which is a form of physical activity). Adopting new rules and new habits could bother you in some way, if you don't make them aware of you. The advantages of the present are those needs to which you find satisfaction, in this case through eating, relaxing and releasing stress. So now ask yourself the following questions:

Why shouldn't I lose weight?

(for example, because eating a lot makes me relax)

So what can I do to keep the need to relax by replacing excessive food consumption?

Or:

Why shouldn't I lose weight?

(for example, because eating a lot helps me relieve stress)

So what can I do to maintain the need to relieve stress by replacing excessive food consumption?

Write these questions in your notebook and answer them ...

5) *Your goal must be ecological, that is to respect your values, your health and your moral ethics.*

The goal must be ecological, but not in the sense of respect for the environment, but rather, of respect due to yourself, your health, your body and your values. If you cut your leg to lose 20 pounds quickly, you would have immediately reached the goal, but you would hurt your body very much and you could even die. In the same way, if you decide not to eat anymore, you will certainly lose a lot of weight, but most likely you will not live long, or if you decide to spend all day running, swimming, playing sports, etc. to lose weight, you will surely lose weight, but you will have to give up all the benefits of your present in which you find satisfaction. All this is not an "ecological" way to achieve your healthy weight. There are, however, many other, much more ecological, ways to achieve the same result.

The 16: 8 DIET that I propose to you in this book is structured to be the most ecological there is, in fact it is simple rules that are based on the physical balance of each of us and on the requests that our body makes to us. The strategies and techniques that you will find can be implemented in total respect of one's moral values and physiological parameters, therefore the method is completely ecological.

Now ask yourself the following questions:

What are the consequences for my health if I lose weight?

What are the consequences for my health if I DO NOT lose weight?

What are the consequences for people around me if I lose weight?

Write these questions in your notebook and answer them ...

Regarding this last question: "What are the consequences for the people around me if I lose weight", a lady told me that her fear was that by losing weight and returning beautiful as she was before, her husband would become "jealous" again ", Because all the men turned to look at her. So she preferred to remain overweight, so nobody looked at her as before and her husband was not jealous, in this way the value of the family she had was safe. Whatever the consequence for those around you, if you lose weight, you must resolve it before starting the weight loss program, otherwise, that will be the cause, conscious or unconscious, for the failure of your goal.

6) Write and declare your goal.

Some time ago, I attended a personal growth course where I learned the big secret to change the way I think and "act": ***the declarations!***

*"What you feel you forget,
remember what you see,
you understand what you do"*

But what is a declaration? The statement is a statement made intensely, out loud. It is a valuable tool. Why? Because everything around us is made up of energy. Energy travels with vibrations and frequencies. Each declaration we make out loud has its own vibration frequency, an energy that vibrates through the cells of our body, and if at the same time we touch a part of our body with one hand, we can perceive its resonance.

The statements convey a powerful message to our unconscious. For this reason, when you get to the end of this chapter I will ask you to do one thing: touch a part of your body with one hand and make a verbal statement. Declaring means officially saying the intention to take a path of action. A statement does not say that a certain thing is true. If I declare: "I am thin, my body is thin", this does not mean that I am really thin, but that I have the intention of becoming or being thin.

This is an acceptable position for our mind, because we are not saying that this is true at the moment, but that it is a projection into the future. We are creating the intention in our mind to be thin. In addition, the statements help us take the necessary actions to turn our intention into reality.

Most people say you have to see it to believe it. Maybe he's right: you have to "see" in our mind, believe in what we "see" in our mind, and then "see" it materialize in real life. Everything that has been created by man has been "seen" before in his mind. The only way to change your "external" world or your body is to change your "internal" world first. It's all very simple: your thoughts lead to your feelings, your feelings lead to your actions, your actions lead to your results.

*Thoughts + Feelings + Actions = **Results!***

This formula is called the "process of manifestation". Have you ever wondered where thoughts come from? Thoughts arise from information "files" stored in the mind. Consequently, just like computers, if we change the programming, the files, we can also change the results. So the first step towards change is awareness. You can't change something in your mind if you don't know it exists first. You must be aware that your mind has a program installed by the system in which we live, a program that has been installed since we were born, first by our parents, then by school and church, then by the people we frequent.

For example, we are all taught to use the right hand as the dominant hand, we use it to write, to eat, to brush our teeth, etc. But this does not mean that we cannot use the left hand better. All of us with a little practice can transfer all the actions we do with the right hand to the left hand, simply by changing our specific mental program on that action.

So if you want to achieve a specific goal, you have to think and act as those who have already achieved that goal think and do. If someone else did it, you can do it too! Let your mind know what you want, imagine it, create it and above all believe it! Then every day you express what you want with your statements. The main reason people don't get what they want is that they don't know what they want; once you've decided what you want, once you've defined your well-formed goal, declare it the right way. This is the way of the warrior. Bankruptcy is not allowed!

"If you want to fly with eagles, don't swim with goslings!"

If you want to become thin and toned, start studying how other people have lost weight, start thinking and acting like them, or simply do what I tell you to do in this book, because it has already been done by thousands of people with excellent results, and if they did it, you can do it too!

*"If you keep doing what you've always done,
you will continue to be what you have always been "*

You already know your way of doing and thinking, now learn to change. My aim is to teach you something new, something different, think differently, act differently to get different results. Now is the time to act! Complete, by writing in your notebook, your goal in the form of a declaration and read it aloud, touching your body with one hand (for example, you can put your right hand on the left side of your chest).

DECLARATION

I .... (write your name)

I want to weigh ...... (write how much you want to weigh)

by .... (write the precise date),

and I really strive to achieve this!

I really strive to become skinny and toned!

Signature………………………………………..

Remember that the order of priorities to achieve your goal is:

BE, DO, HAVE.

If you want to become thin, you must BE Lean in your mind first. Then you have to DO the right actions to become lean (train your mind, train your body, eat properly) and then have a lean and toned body.

What if I can't achieve my goal?

If the fear of failing is a reality for you, know that even if you do not reach your goal, you will still be able to improve your body considerably. Fear is the number one reason why few people set themselves a goal. They unconsciously believe that if they have no goals, they have no way of failing, but they do not understand that they will never succeed in anything, we are all afraid, afraid of making mistakes, afraid of changing, afraid of moving away from someone, fear, fear, fear ...

If you are going to lose 40 pounds in a year, but at the end of the year you have lost "only" 20, it means that you have not reached the goal you had set yourself, but you have still improved your physique significantly. So your efforts have been worthwhile anyway. That's why I ask you to aim for the stars and then fall on top of the mountain ... if you want to lose 40 pounds, then aim to lose 60 pounds, so bad it goes, you will lose 30-40, it is your "real" goal will be achieved . The harder the challenge, the better you will learn to set new standards for yourself.

If you think weight loss is really demanding and complicated, then ask yourself the following question: will you be more successful if you pursue a goal using a strategy that works, or not? To you the judgment. The basic principle is to set a goal and to fight to achieve it, sometimes you will be able to achieve it by respecting your timetable, sometimes it will take you longer than expected, other times you will not get what you set, the important thing is continue to plan and commit, do not give up, you will see that you will reach the finish line. We humans continually tend to get better or worse. If you bought this book and have already written your goal, then it means that you have decided to improve and get better, this is fantastic! If your motivation is strong enough, you can find ways to do practically anything, if your "why" is great, you can find any "how".

"If your motivation is strong enough, you can find ways to do practically anything, if your" why "is great, you can find any" how "..."

Whatever you want to achieve, whether it's a new car, a new home or losing weight, you must always be determined to do it.

"The best thing about the past is that it's gone.

The best thing about the present is that it is a gift.

The best thing about the future is that it is yet to come. "

THE VISION TABLE

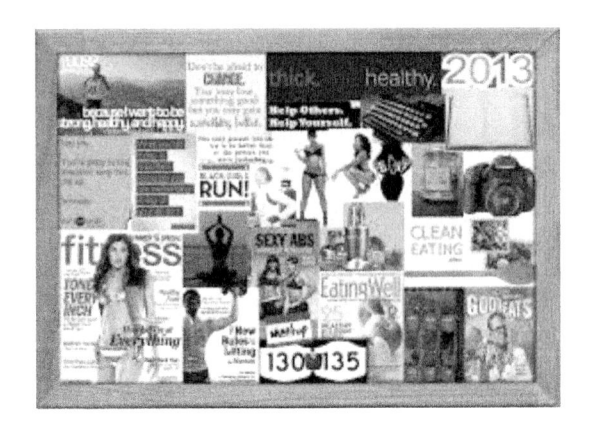

*People complain
because the motivation doesn't last.
If that's why not even a shower,
that's why we do it every day.*

Now let's give physicality to this goal and create your Vision Table.

For this exercise you need some material: scissors, glue, markers, large cardboard, photos cut from color magazines. You can search for photos of places you would like to visit or activities you would like to do when you are in shape. Look for photos where you appear happy (only the face). Clippings from magazines and brochures of bodies you like and other images that represent your goals (in addition to weight loss), such as health, energy, happiness, love ...

Stick photos and images onto the cardboard panel or sheet. Replace the faces of the models with pictures of yourself. Don't worry if they seem strange or disproportionate; the main purpose is to have a clear view of yourself with the body shape you want, all on one page. Add quotes or phrases that inspire you and that can be motivating (In this book you will find many).

Add whatever inspires you: small glued objects, spangles, rhinestones. Write your goal and its deadline clearly, write why you want it, what values or beliefs can help you achieve it.

Let's take an example:

I .... (write your name)

I want to weigh ...... (write your weight)

by .... (write the precise date),

and I really strive to achieve this!

I really strive to become thin and toned because I will like you more, I will feel healthier, I will take the stairs out of breath, I will be able to wear what I want, *(add what you want ...)*

Signature..

Take all the time you need to create this billboard and make it special. This is your vision table. Put what you want! Make it beautiful and then hang it so that it is visible every day. Look at it every day and imagine the feelings you will have when you reach your goal.

The law of focused attention tells us that if there is something you really want to achieve or have in your life, you must behave as if you already have it. So I advise you to go out and buy a new piece of clothing of the size you would like to bring. This will represent the goal you want to reach, hang it outside your wardrobe or near the vision table, where you can often see it. This visual anchor will help you stay on course towards achieving your goal. Every time you step in front of it and see it, stop for a moment and pay attention to the positive feelings, the images of how wonderfully good you will feel and how fantastic you will look when you are able to wear it.

It is essential, for your success, that you identify yourself with all the experiences you have included in your Vision Table: you who wear that new item of clothing, you who run in the park, you who move safely ...

Close your eyes and imagine those scenes ... then enlarge the images as if you were in front of a cinema screen ... increase the brightness of the scene ... increase the sound of the noises or voices around you ... increase the intensity of the colors ...

Do this visualization exercise every day.

GET A VISUAL REPRESENTATION OF WHAT YOU ARE DOING.

If you have to lose 40 pounds, every time you lose a pound create a visual testimony to your success. For example, you can take a bag that can fill up with 40 pounds of sand or salt and every time you lose a pound, fill that bag with a pound of sand or salt. When you lose 40 pounds and fill the sack with 40 pounds of sand or salt, that sack will serve as a reminder of how much extra weight you carried. This visual representation will help you not to regain that extra useless weight and to keep the goal achieved.

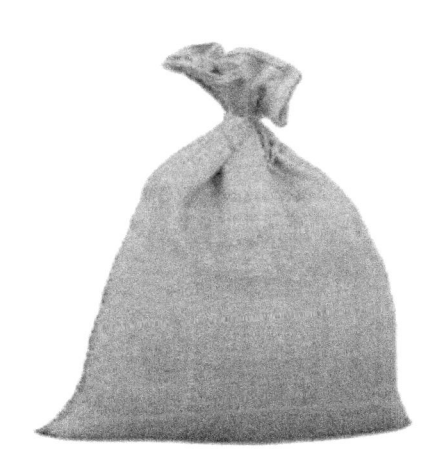

Chapter 1
Let's start from the basics (Chronoalimentation)

"If you're going to lose weight, don't wait for it to happen, make it happen, be patient and believe it."

Developed in recent years by an Italian doctor, Mauro Todisco (who by the way is one of the doctors who follow Dr. Di Bella), chronological nutrition has proved to be the most effective trend for optimal nutritional intake. But in this case it is not the usual bizarre diet, which every now and then is in fashion, but a real science based on precise hormonal cycles.

The chronological diet is based on the principle that our hormonal flows are significantly different throughout the day and therefore the quality of the food has different values depending on the time of intake. But let's see, point by point, the action and hourly activity of hormones that can significantly influence the distribution of our meals. Let's start with insulin: insulin is a hormone produced by the pancreas and among its many functions, the main one is to allow the entry of glucose into the cells. It can be considered a decidedly fattening hormone as it allows fat cells to produce triglycerides (practically 85% of subcutaneous storage fats), while blocking the enzyme that splits them and starting what produces the storage of fats. It also helps transform glucose into additional fatty acids.

Cortisonic hormones are secreted by the adrenal glands, they also have many functions but the most interesting for our purposes seems to be to increase the level of glucose in the blood. They act in the sugar transport mechanism inside the cell and in the decrease of its use. These actions can create an increase in the cleavage of triglycerides and consequently of fatty acids that cortisone hormones can then use as energy instead of the classic glucose. In practice these hormones counteract insulin in its action of using glucose for our adipose panniculus. They are at the highest level in the morning (most likely to prepare the body for daily activity), they remain very high even until the early afternoon, and then gradually descend to the night minimum.

The hormones T3 and T4 are produced by the thyroid and perform a fundamental function on our metabolism, above all influencing the speed of assimilation of food. The higher their values, the greater the ability to convert food into energy and not fat. The T3 reaches its maximum level around 1 pm and the T4 at 4 pm.

"The T3 reaches its maximum level around 1pm and the T4 at 4pm ..."

Remember this information well, because it is in these 4 hours that you can eat your favorite food, especially carbohydrates (pasta, desserts, etc.).

Growth hormone, on the other hand, peaks in the first two hours after falling asleep. Secreted by the pituitary gland, it has remarkably interesting functions as regards the lean mass / fat mass ratio. This hormone, whose main peculiarity is precisely that of making all organs grow in the developmental age, also allows in adulthood to stimulate the use of fats and the increase in muscle mass. This occurs because the poly-peptide activates the enzyme that promotes the cleavage of the deposit triglycerides, using them for energy purposes and in the meantime reducing the use of glucose. It also limits the transformation of amino acids into glucose and increases protein production. In practice, it makes you lose weight only of fat without losing muscle forms: just what we want. Growth hormone levels remain very high up to the age of twenty, then progressively decrease to the age of thirty, from where a further drop occurs.

To naturally stimulate the increase in the hormone, **the use of good amounts of protein at dinner** (the meal closest to night rest) **and the almost total elimination of carbohydrates can be successfully used**, as they interfere with the peak GH night. The association of carbohydrates and proteins with meals can also increase the pancreas secretion of insulin by double. **Meals should therefore be dissociated.**

So as you may have understood there are 3 simple rules to respect to burn fat naturally respecting the hormonal cycles of your body:

1) Carbohydrates from 13 to 16

2) Protein at dinner

3) Dissociate meals

Now you will ask yourself. What about breakfast?

Calmly, soon I'll tell you what to do for breakfast ...

To complete the picture, we must finally explain that there are two fundamental overweight somatotypes: **the android and the gynoid.**

The android type, which mainly characterizes men, has fat accumulated especially in the upper body. The most affected sections are: the abdomen, torso, shoulders and neck. Main responsible for this distribution are male hormones, androgens, which present in a higher than normal way in women, can cause the same type of overweight. To predispose this accumulation of subcutaneous fats are the cortisone hormones, which in the androids are particularly high. As we have already seen, these hormones, by transforming amino acids into glucose, can, if above normal, predispose to fattening.

The hypothalamus, the gland that controls the pituitary gland to produce corticosteroids, however, can be inhibited by two neurotransmitters, norepinephrine and GABA. Since the precursors of these two substances are produced from three amino acids, namely phenylalanine / tyrosine (norepinephrine) and glutamic acid (GABA), to curb the excessive production of corticosteroids, a good amount of protein must be consumed. On the other hand, another neurotransmitter, serotonin, which increases its concentration with the intake of carbohydrates, has instead a stimulating function on the hypothalamus. So for the android the moral is: **less carbohydrates and more proteins.**

In the "gynoid" overweight, the fat is distributed in the lower abdomen, in the upper part of the thighs, in the buttocks and in the hips. It is due to the action of female hormones and therefore women suffer most. To understand how we can fight it, it is useful to make a small digression on the functioning of our nervous system.

The central one controls all the voluntary functions of our body, that is, the movements that we command with conscious thought. Instead, the autonomic nervous system presides over involuntary functions such as maintaining body temperature, sweating, heart rate, stomach, intestines and metabolism.

All these functions take place without us realizing it. The autonomous is composed of two sections in antagonism with each other: the sympathetic nervous system and the parasympathetic. In general, the sympathetic promotes physical and mental work while the parasympathetic saves and stores energy when there is no intense effort. In addition to other functions, the sympathetic reduces the secretion of insulin, allows the splitting of the triglycerides accumulated in the subcutaneous and accelerates the metabolism. The parasympathetic instead optimizes the accumulation of storage fats, increases the secretion of insulin and the assimilation of nutrients. It is logical that this continuous struggle between the two sections, depending on the prevalence of one or the other, allows for higher or lower metabolism. Normally during the day the sympathetic prevails while at night the parasympathetic dominates. **In practice, you must eat abundantly during the day and make a more contained dinner in order not to help the accumulation of fats.**

Ginoid obesity is therefore normally characterized by excessive parasympathetic activity. Let's go now to see how to act at the level of the hypothalamus (the gland that underlies the functioning of all the other hormonal functions), to optimize the metabolism. The hypothalamus is strongly influenced by two nuclei; the ventromedial nucleus, which has the function of stimulating the sympathetic system to cleave the deposit triglycerides and the ventrolateral nucleus which predisposes the parasympathetic to deposit the fats. Serotonin, which as mentioned above increases with the intake of carbohydrates, stimulates the activity of the ventromedial nucleus which has a function exactly opposite to the ventrolateral one. The latter is thus hampered and consequently reduces its fattening action. **For "ginoids", therefore, the carbohydrate quota should not be kept low, provided that the principles of chrono-feeding are still followed.**

In summary, to keep the body fat level low and at the same time not to lose muscle forms (always remember that a beautiful body must be thin but shaped, with beautiful shapes) you must:

• *Consume carbohydrates in the first part of the day so that the highest cortisone hormones counteract the fattening action of insulin, thus storing all glucose in more useful glycogen. The most abundant meal will have to be lunch as at 2 pm and 4 pm there is the peak of the thyroid hormones T3 and T4, which further speed up the metabolism. Carbohydrates should not be taken with protein.*

• *In the evening only meals with proteins without carbohydrates, so as not to interfere with the release of GH.*

In the midst of a lot of nutritional information and types of diets it is easy to lose one's bearings and get confused about the choice of this or that food strategy. However, experience in the field has suggested to me that, as with the various types of training, many times each individual seems to react more or less well to the same food line, moreover one has to deal with the different needs of the subjects; in fact, many diets require some time and a lot of precision in preparing meals that not everyone can (or wants) to have. Not to mention that between the accuracy required by some diets and the attention in the weight of meals, on the whole, many may lose patience!

If you are an overweight subject, with the main goal of losing weight, with limited time available and with little accurate availability of meals (practically most people), chronological nutrition is normally well accepted. The simplicity of application (the fact that there is no control over the weight of the food and the good level of effectiveness) has made it successful in almost all the individuals in which it has been applied. I propose below the two schemes, one for subjects with superfluous "android" fat and one for "ginoids".

The principles of chronological nutrition can be summarized in the following rules of behavior, observing which it is possible to reduce body weight simply by following the biological rhythms of our body.

1) Cereals and their derivatives (bread, pasta, rice, breadsticks, flour, semolina, biscuits, crackers, rusks, oat or corn flakes, etc.) should be consumed in the first part of the day (from 13 to 16). The same rule applies to legumes (chickpeas, beans, lentils, etc.) and potatoes. Lunch must be the most abundant meal of the day. For first courses, at lunch, the quantity not to be exceeded is that contained in the internal circle of a normal serving dish. Bread can be eaten for lunch; however, its consumption should be modest (no more than one slice). No bread for dinner. For lunch you can also eat your favorite dessert.

2) Among carbohydrate-based foods, those subjected to fine division or elimination of fibers are to be avoided. Therefore, cane sugar or honey is preferable to white sugar, and for the same reason to whole grain cereals without bran. Furthermore,

rice and potatoes are more suitable than bread and pasta, which are digested faster.

3) Meat, fish, eggs and dairy products must, alternately, constitute the evening meal (from 19:00 to 20:00). Three times a week, protein foods can also be eaten as a replacement for first courses. For the amount of protein-based foods, especially fish, you can eat it to your satisfaction, obviously do not overdo it ...

4) Vegetables and vegetables can be present in both meals.

5) Seasonal fruit must be eaten by 17:00, you can eat it half an hour before lunch or three hours later, but it must be avoided at dinner. The ideal, however, would be to use it for the afternoon snack, in the latter case, however, preferring the less sugary fruits (pineapple, tangerines, grapefruits, strawberries, cherries, watermelons, peaches, melons, raspberries). The fruit must be introduced whole and not in the form of juices or juices. Canned fruit should be avoided.

6) The consumption of wine and beer should be avoided at lunchtime, a moderate intake (a glass) of these drinks, if it is appreciated, is instead allowed to eat mainly protein in the evening, as alcohol facilitates the digestion of proteins.

7) The condiments should not be used excessively, but neither should they be abolished; vegetable fats (especially olive oil) should be preferred over animal fats such as butter, lard and lard.

8) The menus must be varied and appetizing: there is no need to go hungry, there are no penalties to be served; the worst enemy of weight loss is boredom (and repetitiveness).

9) It may be useful to have some coffee during the morning but without sweetener and not after meals containing carbohydrates. Wine, beer and coffee should never be combined with carbohydrates

A Chrono-power supply: Android type limenti e Orario di assunzione	
Cereals and derivatives	from 13 to 16
Legumes potatoes	from 13 to 16
Meat Fish 3 times a week You can also eat eggs for lunch Dairy products instead of carbohydrates	from 19 to 20
Carrots Dried mushrooms Artichokes Beets broccoli Brussels sprouts verze Rape tomatoes	from 13 to 14
Other vegetables	from 13 to 20
Bananas Grapes Figs persimmons chestnuts Dried fruit	These fruits, if possible, for the Android type are to be avoided
Other fruit	no later than 5pm

A Chrono-feeding: Ginoid type limenti e Orario di assunzione	
Cereals and derivatives	from 13 to 16
Legumes potatoes	from 13 to 16
Meat Fish eggs dairy product	from 19 to 20
carrots Dried mushrooms Artichokes Beets Broccoli Brussels sprouts Verza Rape tomatoes	from 13 to 16
Other vegetables	from 13 to 20
Bananas Grapes Figs persimmon chestnuts Dried fruit	no later than 4pm
Other fruit	no later than 5pm

Chapter 2
16: 8 DIET: The Secret Formula for Weight Loss

"To change your body it is essential to change your mind."

A few years ago, surfing the web, I read a "new and fascinating" theory concerning the way of eating.

This theory appeared in contrast to the advice that often circulates in the fitness environment and in opposition to some guidelines of proper nutrition.

Some of the principles that were contested were, for example, the following:

• *Better to eat little and often (essential to keep the metabolism "active")*

• *Don't skip breakfast*

• *Make "a king's breakfast, a queen's lunch and a poor dinner"*

• *Do not skip meals (it would be harmful to health)*

• *Do not fast (metabolism would "slow down" and induce protein catabolism)*

• *Eat often to avoid sudden changes in blood sugar*

* *Do not exceed with proteins (their rate of assimilation is limited)*

* *Do not train on an empty stomach (it would promote muscle catabolism and loss of strength in anaerobic sports)*

This new theory immediately seemed fascinating to me because on that site it was written in black and white that losing weight using that type of diet would greatly limit the loss of muscle mass. So less fat but with a more toned physique!

So I began to study and document myself by reading both the scientific articles shared on the Martin Berkhan website, and by deepening the topic through independent bibliographic research.

So I discovered that this theory-way of feeding is called with the term "16:8 DIET"

Given the numerous scientific evidences in favor of the 16:8 DIET, I thought it was legitimate to ask whether those famous principles were always valid or are they instead of myths or, as often happens, the truth lies in the middle? What could be the best way to disclose them?

The world of gyms and diets as we know is full of false myths, and these myths are kept alive by:

1. Repetition

If something is repeated often enough everyone starts to believe it and becomes the "truth". If everyone says the same thing, it must be true. The fact that celebrities from fitness and diets propagate these myths doesn't help. Most people think that if these people say it, it must be true.

2. Commercial interests.

For example, in the supplement sector, the message that eating frequently offers a metabolic advantage is often disseminated, and in doing so, of course, more supplements are purchased. In fact, those who don't have time to prepare and eat six hot meals a day turn to powders that replace meals, smoothies and protein bars. There is no commercial incentive to tell people that three meals a day is more than enough.

3. Poor update.

Updating is essential because in twenty years science has made great strides and it is unthinkable not to ask whether some theories should be confirmed or refuted. In this book, therefore, I wanted to show that the advice that often circulates in the fitness environment and some guidelines for proper nutrition are not the only way to eat healthily and healthily, but that they are only guidelines valid to eat and there are also other methods that should be taken more into consideration, for example: intermittent fasting or 16: 8 DIET

Intermittent fasting (IF) is a diet that alternates 16 hour fasting phases with 8 hour feeding phases.

Intermittent fasting is a fairly easy way to have a calorie restriction, even if it goes against many popular beliefs and nutrition guidelines, such as: eating little and often, skipping breakfast hurts, eating often accelerates the metabolism and not doing it would lower it, eat frequently to prevent the risk of muscle catabolism, etc.

Many of these are not truths, but only tips to prevent excess calories or unregulated nutrition. For example, it has been seen that eating with a diet that has an intermittency between feeding and fasting has a lower loss of lean mass compared to an equivalent in kcal of classic calorie restriction.

And it has been seen that in normocaloric there is an improvement in body composition, i.e. fat loss and lean mass gain. Perhaps the reason can be found in hormonal / physiological changes.

• Fasting causes an increase in GH levels, the latter promotes lipolysis and the release of fatty acids from adipocytes.
• Fasting reduces insulin levels and improves their sensitivity, insulin inhibits lipolysis.
• Fasting causes an increase in adrenaline and norepinephrine, which increase energy expenditure in short-term fasting, also activate lipase, a sensitive hormone present in adipose tissue by stimulating the release of body fat.

Eating often does not speed up the metabolism, there are many studies that prove it. This myth perhaps arose from the misinterpretation of the diet-induced thermogenesis, whenever we eat we paradoxically have an energy expenditure to digest and absorb food, this metabolic rate is different for proteins, carbohydrates or fats ... this energy expenditure is proportional to the quantity of the ingested KCALs.

So 2000kcal eaten in 1 or 3 or 9 meals always have the same metabolic rate.

Popular beliefs say that eating a lot in the evening makes you fat. There are no controlled studies showing where larger meals if eaten in the evening have a negative influence on body composition.

People who eat late at night, like snacking in front of the TV, probably weigh more, but it is not the fact that they eat at night, but their lifestyle that is wrong. There are studies that say the exact opposite of popular beliefs, there seems to be an improvement in body composition in a calorie restriction if more abundant meals, especially based on proteins, are eaten in the evening.

Short-term fasting up to a maximum of 16 hours as recommended in intermittent fasting does not cause a decrease in the metabolic rate, but rather a slight increase due to adrenaline and norepinephrine.

Only after 60 hours there is a reduction in the metabolic rate.

Intermittent fasting does not necessarily require fasting training. However, it has been seen that strength and low intensity endurance training are not affected after a short fast. And there are studies that show better resting concentrations of muscle glycogen after a fasting workout.

Remember: *One of the rules for being free is to question everything. If there is something that attracts you and you want to try, try it. If something sounds crazy to you, ask yourself why you think it sounds crazy, and do your own research and experiment it before you have any prejudices and condemn it.*

This is what I did, I did a scientific research, I talked about it with a friend of mine, a dietician, I tried it first on myself (with excellent results), then my friend a dietician extended the test on his patients, and the results were crazy, people were happy because they lost weight but were not hungry, because after the 16-hour fast, of which not to forget that 8 hours of fasting are night, after I said, from 13 to 16 they could eat practically that they wanted (pasta, pizza, sweets, etc.) and this on a psychological level did not make the diet a problem, also I remind you that after 21 days everyone got used to not eating for breakfast, everyone, and everyone after these 21 days during morning they said they felt more energetic, active and mentally lucid ...

What are the disadvantages of intermittent fasting?

In my experience, I have found very few side effects with intermittent fasting.

The biggest problem I have found, and the biggest concern that most people have, is that intermittent fasting will lead to low energy, little mental lucidity and immense fear of starving during the fasting period. People are worried that they will be unhappy all morning because they have not eaten any food, and therefore their job, or any other task they will have to do, will be inefficient.

Yes, the initial transition from EAT WHEN YOU WANT, to intermittent fasting can be a bit of a jolt to the system. However, once the transition days (21 days) are exceeded, your body will quickly adapt to learning how to function just as well by eating only a few times a day.

"So why do I feel bad when I skip breakfast?"

In my humble opinion, a good part of the bad mood is the result of eating habits. If you eat every three hours, your body will begin to have an appetite every three hours because it has become so used to it. If you eat breakfast every morning, your body expects to eat food as soon as you wake up.

It is only a self-conviction.

Once your body no longer expects food all day, every day (or in the morning), these side effects will become less of a problem (thanks to a substance that our body produces called ghrelin).

Think about it, how could cave dwellers survive without having refrigerators and supermarkets available? We have certainly found ways to survive during times of abundance and famine. It actually takes around 84 hours of fasting before glucose levels are adversely affected. We are talking about small fasts (16 hours), so it does not concern us.

An important warning:

Intermittent fasting can be complex for people who have problems with blood sugar regulation, suffer from hypoglycemia, or have diabetes. If you fall into this category, I highly recommend that you consult your doctor or nutritionist before setting up your feeding schedule. I believe that more research needs to be done for these particular cases and therefore I advise you to do what works best for you.

Why it works.

Although we know that not all calories are created equal, calorie restriction plays a central role in weight loss. When you fast (for 16 hours a day), you are also limiting your calorie intake more easily over the week. This will give your body a chance to lose weight because it is simply eating fewer calories than it was before.

Because it simplifies your day.

Instead of having to prepare, pack, eat your meals every 2-3 hours, simply skip a meal or two and only worry about eating the food in the feeding window (8 hours). It takes less time (and potentially money). Instead of having to prepare 3-6 meals a day, you only need to prepare two of them. Instead of stopping what you're doing six times a day, simply stop and eat only twice. Rather than having to do the dishes six times, you just have to do them twice. Instead of buying six meals a day, you only need to buy two.

How to start?

Having said that, what you simply have to do at the beginning is to continue eating everything you ate before but only from 13:00 to 21:00. While from 21:00 to 13:00 you don't have to eat anything.

Why exactly these times?

Because in the morning our body is in a catabolic phase and fasting helps our body to "detoxify" from the food we took the day before, while from 13:00 to 16:00 it is the best time to take carbohydrates, for hormones T3 and T4 which are produced by the thyroid and perform a fundamental function on our metabolism, above all influencing the speed of assimilation of food. The higher their values, the greater the ability to convert food into energy and not fat.

While in the evening, before 21:00, the ideal would be to eat protein accompanied by vegetables to stimulate GH. GH or growth hormone peaks in the first two hours after falling asleep. Secreted by the pituitary gland, it has remarkably interesting functions as regards the lean mass / fat mass ratio.

This hormone, whose main peculiarity is precisely that of making all organs grow in the developmental age, also allows in adulthood to stimulate the use of fats and the increase in lean body mass. This occurs because the poly-peptide activates the enzyme that promotes the cleavage of the deposit triglycerides, using them for energy purposes and in the meantime reducing the use of glucose.

It also limits the transformation of amino acids into glucose and increases protein production. In practice, it makes you lose weight only of fat without losing muscle forms: just what we want.

Here is an example of an ideal day of intermittent fasting feeding:

- From 9:00 pm to 1:00 pm drink only water, tea or herbal tea without sugar
- From 13:00 to 16:00 eat what you like, bread, pasta, sweets, etc. obviously without overdoing it (this also helps you on a psychological level not to perceive intermittent fasting as a restriction)

- In the afternoon until 17:00 if you get hungry, eat some fruit
- Before 21:00 make dinner with proteins: meat or fish (to be preferred) to combine with vegetables, or cheeses always with vegetables.

As you can see, in principle it is not a complicated diet and you don't have to give up your favorite food, but I assure you that it works great!

But wait it doesn't end here, this is just the beginning ...

What you have just finished reading is a powerful food strategy that will make you lose many kilograms alone, but there are small tricks that can even double the speed to lose fat!

Chapter 3

Are you hungry ... or are you thirsty? Water: the secret of 16.8 DIET for weight loss in a healthy and fast way

"Alcohol hurts, but water does even worse: it kills you if you don't drink it!"

(Jaume Perich)

If you don't drink the right amount of water daily, your body cannot transform fat into energy and you struggle to lose weight even if you eat less.

The body is made up of cells, which like us need food, water and oxygen. If these things are provided to them, they manage to work well and therefore are also able to take fat, use it as food and turn it into energy.

For you this means losing fat, weight, centimeters and feeling more energetic.

Interesting right?

Do you think that water is so important for cells that dehydration of only 1% of body weight affects the physical activities of our body. If dehydration rises to 5%, cramps, weakness and increased irritability appear. With 10% there is a risk of heat stroke, and survival itself begins to be endangered. 20%

dehydration can lead to risk of death due to complete arrest of physiological functions.

An athlete who does exercise puts his body in a dehydration situation of only 2% reduces the performance by 20%. Even if the water content in the cell drops below 50%, the vital processes become paralyzed, often even irreversibly.

Why do I tell you this? Because I want you to begin to understand that if there is not the right water, your cells cannot work! If they don't work, your whole body doesn't work well, it doesn't "respond to commands". If you are on a diet or rather if you intend to follow the diet of this course, you will make many sacrifices and extra effort, if you do not drink the right amount of water for you.

The cause of many diseases that currently afflict millions of people around the world is due to the fact that we do not drink enough water. Diseases like asthma, diabetes, arthritis, angina, cholesterol, Alzheimer's, hypertension, etc., including obesity, are all consequences of dehydration of our body.

This is the revolutionary medical discovery of an Iranian doctor, Fereydoon Batmanghelidj, he says that many degenerative diseases could be prevented simply by drinking more water daily ...

Everyone knows that water is "good" for the body, but few know how important it is for everyone's well-being or what happens to the body if it does not receive its daily water requirement.

A mistake that many make, and that of thinking that tea, coffee, alcohol and soft drinks such as fruit juices or even worse than carbonated and sugary drinks, can be substitutes for water, even if those drinks contain water, in reality they contain also diuretic and dehydrating elements, such as caffeine.

Then the water contained in them is expelled with urine, causing another thirst stimulus, and as long as you continue drinking sweet drinks, your body will always be thirsty ...

When you are thirsty, your body wants water, only water!

Having said that, do you know why obese people are always on the rise?

Because they don't know how to distinguish hunger from thirst and they don't know the difference between liquids and water ...

the central control system of the brain recognizes when the available energy levels are too low for its functioning.

The feelings of hunger and thirst both arise from low energy levels, they are generated simultaneously to indicate the needs of the brain.

If we do not recognize the feeling of thirst, we interpret both signals as a stimulus to eat.

We also eat when our body is actually thirsty ...

people who drink water half an hour before meals and 2-3 hours after meals, manage to separate the two thirst-hunger sensations. In this way, having the body always hydrated, they do not overeat to satisfy, in "reality", the need to take water.

This means losing weight simply by drinking "before" being thirsty, the reason why we tend to gain weight is simple: we eat to provide energy to the brain for its incessant activity, but only 20% of that food reaches the brain.

The rest is stored, unless you do physical activity or have a job that makes you consume the remaining 80%.

While when the source of energy is water, there is no deposit of fat, excess water is simply disposed of in the form of urine.

Your body has an absolute need to take at least eight 250 cc glasses of water a day, obviously alcohol, coffee and drinks that contain sugars do not count as water.

Even better is if you decide not to drink them at all!

To know the right amount of water for you, some experts recommend doing this simple calculation:

weight x 3: 100 = Water needed

Do the calculation right away. What's your weight? Multiply by 3, divide by 100. How much water should you drink? If you are already drinking it, congratulations! You are on the right track and if you are still not getting results it is because you probably need to review how you feed yourself ...

If, on the other hand, you are not doing it, you are probably thinking that it is difficult for you to reach the right amount of water, because you do not feel the urge to thirst, because you are often out and about for work, etc.

The best times to drink water are at least a glass half an hour before meals and a glass 2-3 hours after meals, plus two more glasses during the day. Obviously this is the minimum amount you should drink. The ideal would be around 2.5 liters per day or in any case the quantity that came out of the previous mathematical calculation.

Here are some tips to help you drink more:

1) Start with a half-liter bottle in the morning as soon as you wake up then another half-liter bottle in the afternoon, do this for a week and you will see that you will already start feeling better ... then gradually increase by adding another bottle half an hour before of lunch and after a few days another in the evening half an hour before dinner. Get organized right away by putting bottles everywhere: in the car, at work and at home. Put one on the desk, one near the sofa, one in the kitchen in plain sight, etc ...

2) Remember not to drink during meals, so as not to dilute the gastric juices involved in digestion, but always remember to drink half an hour before in order to alleviate hunger.

3) Try to drink a little water at a time, but often, because drinking all the water in a single moment is useless. Better a sip every hour than a liter all at once. If you drink a liter of water in a row, your body cannot use it all at once, so after 5 minutes you will have to run to the bathroom. Otherwise if you drink it a little at a time your body will be able to absorb it and use it to make your body work better and therefore also to lose weight faster.

With increasing water intake, the thirst mechanism becomes more efficient. By regulating water intake according to meal times, blood is prevented from thickening as a result of food intake.

But what water should I drink?

Let's start by saying that you have to drink natural water and not carbonated water, because 2.5 liters of carbonated water a day would swell your stomach like a balloon.

Some find it difficult to digest even natural water, this depends on the fixed residue of the water (i.e. the mineral salts and other substances contained in it).

On the label of the various brands of water you will find the word residual fixed at 180 °, the lower the value, the more digestible the water. I advise you to choose water with a value between 50 milligrams and 500 milligrams per liter. Obviously the closer you get to 50 milligrams, the better ...

What happens to you if you drink less than the amount of water your body needs?

You may feel tired, you realize it when you go to the beach, usually in the evening you feel tired and without strength. This depends on the fact that sun, sweat and wind have taken away a lot of water from your body.

You may have difficulty concentrating.

You could almost certainly suffer from constipation (I remind you that normalcy is "going to the bathroom" 1 or 2 times a day).

From an aesthetic point of view, the skin may appear dull and dry.

And if you are a woman you are likely to have water retention problems. (in fact, when you don't give your body what little it has, it tends to "keep it").

Your body cannot detoxify well so you may have pain, headaches, and other minor ailments.

But what are the symptoms of dehydration?

-One of the most common symptoms is chronic fatigue.

-You may have difficulty concentrating.

-You may have water retention problems.

-Your skin becomes dry and dull.

-You may suffer from constipation.

- Back and joint pains due to lack of lubrication ...

I could go on ... but I think it is enough for you to start drinking WATER now!

Do not wait, immediately drink a glass of water, take the healthy habit of drinking as I explained in this chapter, you will see that one day you will thank me. I have already done it with those who taught me to drink 2.5 liters of water per day as a minimum quantity and to drink it half an hour before meals and two to three hours after meals.

I swear to you that if you do, only this chapter will help you lose a lot of weight, it will help you eat less, but above all it will help you feel better in health.

"Water is the least expensive form of medicine for a dehydrated body"

But let's also see what happens to you when you drink the right amount of water. Remember that most of our body is made up of water such as:

• Blood is made up of 85% water. Drinking water will improve your circulation, which means: a better flow of oxygen, a better supply of nutrients to all organs, and a better elimination of waste and toxins.
• The brain is made up of 75% water. Drinking water will make you mentally clearer.
• Our joints need to be lubricated. Drinking water will make you lose some "aches or pains" and will protect you from joint problems.
• Our body needs water to perform all its functions, including that of making you lose weight.

Now I want you to read a study from the University of Washington that says:

-A glass of water takes away the feeling of hunger at night for almost 100% of people on a diet.

-Lack of water is the No. 1 factor in the cause of fatigue during the day.

- Preliminary studies indicate that 8 to 10 glasses of water per day could significantly alleviate back and joint pain in 80% of people suffering from these ailments.

-A simple 2% reduction in water in the human body can cause short-term memory inconsistency, math problems, and difficulty focusing on the computer screen or a printed page.

-Drinking 8 glasses of water a day decreases the risk of colon cancer by 45%, can reduce the risk of breast cancer by 79% and the probability of it developing in the bladder by 50%.

So, as incredible as it may seem, water is probably the most effective element for weight loss. While people are constantly looking for the magic thermogenic that helps them "burn fat", the safest and equally effective alternative can be found on the tap at home or on supermarket shelves.

How is it possible? The reasons are manifold. First of all, water has an anorectic effect, that is, it reduces the appetite stimulus in a natural way. Secondly, the water helps the body to metabolize the accumulated fat allowing a better functioning of the liver and kidneys.

In fact, if you don't take a sufficient amount of water, your kidneys don't work properly. And when the kidneys don't work well, part of their function is done by the liver. One of the main functions of the liver is to metabolize part of the stored fat and transform it into energy that can be used by our body.

But if the liver is engaged in fulfilling the functions of the kidneys, it cannot perform its specific metabolic functions at full capacity. As a result, the liver metabolizes less fat and fat accumulates in the body, preventing weight loss.

Drinking plenty of water also increases the frequency of urinations. Urination and sweating are two ways in which the body dissipates heat (energy / calories). Increasing the number of urinations means dispersing more calories and therefore giving more calories to the environment.

Some experts have speculated that drinking cold water allows you to consume more calories because the body must use more energy to heat the water. However, the data available are still too few and the differences in the results obtained by the researchers with their studies on increasing energy expenditure for 60 minutes - ranging from 4.5% to 24% - suggest the need for further research.

Instead, it has been verified how water-induced thermogenesis can be attributable to the effect it has on the sympathetic nervous system. Although the process has not yet been fully understood, researchers have found that taking large quantities of water increases sympathetic nerve activity and the release of norepinephrine which, in turn, increases the conversion of glycogen into glucose and stimulates the lipolysis.

In practice, drinking water helps stimulate the metabolism and consume more calories!

What if I love to drink coffee?

If you love drinking coffee and don't want to do without it, then immediately after your usual cup of coffee, drink an extra glass of water immediately, because coffee contributes to the dehydration of the body. The same trick applies to alcohol.

Water and lemon

Another tip that I want to give you is to drink a cup of lukewarm water every morning on an empty stomach (I recommend, I said lukewarm, not too hot, because excessive heat disperses vitamin C), with half a squeezed lemon. In this way you will not only stimulate the digestive system, but you will also enjoy a series of benefits for your health:

• helps fight colds during the winter thanks to its vitamin C content
• regulates blood pressure
• reduces the general acidity level of the body helping you lose weight faster
• helps fight hunger attacks thanks to its rich pectin content
• promotes the production of bile by helping digestion
• promotes urination and therefore the expulsion of toxins
• reduces skin imperfections and wrinkles
• can relieve gingivitis and toothache and keep the breath fresh

In short, we can say that lemon is healthy and beneficial and drinking it in the morning with water can only help to prevent or resolve some ailments that affect daily well-being.

Chapter 4
Green Tea, a Superdrink for burning fat

"The way to heaven goes through a teapot."

(English proverb)

This chapter will be dedicated to a Superdrink: green tea.

I would like to highlight the benefits and characteristics of this ancient drink of a thousand virtues (the first green tea drinker was a Chinese emperor in 2700 BC), in the hope that you can appreciate its value and choose to include some cups of green tea in the food program .

The green tea leaves that have always been used, especially in the East, as health carriers can be considered as a miraculous natural medicine.

All tea varieties are made from a single plant: the Camelia Sinensis. The difference between the various types (black tea, green tea, white tea, red tea etc ...) is due to the subsequent oxidation treatment to which the leaves of this plant are subjected.

Although today's English culture classifies tea into at least 5 categories, traditionally there are only three types of tea, namely: black tea, oolong tea and green tea.

The names with which tea is usually identified refer to the region of origin of the plant, for example: Ceylon, Darjeeling, Souchong, etc ...

The tea varieties are classified according to the processing method and the duration of the fermentation of the leaves.

Black tea is dried and fermented; partially fermented oolong tea; while green tea is simply washed and heated to prevent fermentation and is therefore immediately ready for use.

Green tea is obtained through a vaporization process of fresh tea leaves and this is the reason why green tea contains about 40% of polyphenol, a flavonoid compound, which makes it somewhat nutritious and healthy for your body.

Green tea effectively helps your body burn calories and fat by increasing your metabolic rate.

Have you ever heard of epigallocatechin?

Epigallocatechin is a chemical compound present in large quantities in green tea. This compound allows weight loss, collaborates with the metabolism in burning excess calories and fat. Other substances contained in green tea such as tea flavine and rubigine tea have the ability to fight fats.

Many studies show that including green tea in your diet is of great help in promoting weight loss.

There is no single food or miraculous substance that can make you lose weight but integrating 2/3 cups a day of green tea into your food program has proven to be an effective technique capable of making you lose weight in a healthy and natural way thanks to the action diuretic and lipolytic properties of this drink. In fact, taking green tea will cause all the impurities accumulated by eating to be expelled through urine and will therefore be of great help to combat water retention, to solve cellulite problems and to lose excess pounds.

Green tea amplifies the sense of satiety, acts as a calming of the digestive organs, promotes purification and is rich in minerals and vitamins.

What does green tea contain?

• a cup of green tea is made up of 90% water;
• depending on the varieties, green tea is rich in vitamin C / B / K / A / D / E / H;
• a cup of green tea has no calories;
• green tea contains precious minerals for your body including: magnesium / zinc / aluminum / chromium and selenium;
• green tea is rich in tannins, flavonoids and polyphenols, including epigallocatechin with known antioxidant (and therefore anti-aging) properties;
• although in small quantities, green tea contains caffeine.

Some studies conducted in Japan show that green tea helps to burn calories through thermogenesis: a particular metabolic process that consists in the production of heat by the body, especially in fat and muscle tissue.

Remember, however, that the fundamentals for disposing of excess pounds and maintaining your healthy weight are: mental attitude, nutrition education and physical activity. So to get concrete results I recommend you integrate green tea with a healthy and balanced diet and regular physical activity.

Here are some lines from an interview by Oprah Winfrey with Dr. Nicholas Perricone (doctor of medicine, specialized in dermatology and nutritionist recognized worldwide as an expert in the field of anti-aging).

Oprah: *Now I've read in your book that you said if I just replaced coffee with green tea instead, that I could lose 10 pounds in six weeks.*

Dr. Perricone: *Absolutely.*

Oprah: *Now really. How could that be -- what is the big deal about this?*

Dr. Perricone: *Coffee has organic acids that raise your blood sugar, raise insulin. Insulin puts a lock on body fat. When you switch over to green tea, you get your caffeine, you're all set, but you will drop your insulin levels and body fat will fall very rapidly. So 10 pounds (4.5 kg) in six weeks, I will guarantee it.*

Oprah: *I'm gonna do that. OK. That is so good! Wow! That is great.*

Adapted from:

The Oprah Winfrey Show: "Look 10 Years Younger in 10 Days" -- Nov. 10, 2004.

It has been shown that lemon promotes the absorption of the catechins contained in green tea, therefore adding a few drops of lemon to your green tea increases the beneficial effects of the drink. Furthermore, a drop of lemon can make the taste of green tea more pleasant even if I assure you that it is also delicious natural!

To fully enjoy all the beneficial effects, to preserve the antioxidants and nutritional values of green tea, it is best to drink it immediately after the infusion.

Here are some tips for making an excellent cup of green tea:

• first you need a teapot, green tea is dry and compact but needs to expand when infused. So the strainers are not good, they are too small;
• heat the water to about 90 degrees, the water must not boil;
• pour the water into the teapot and let it rest for a few seconds, in this way the temperature will drop to 80 degrees. Perfect temperature for green tea!
• uses good quality water;
• use about 6 grams of tea for every 50 ml of water;
• to obtain a light taste, leave to infuse for about 3/4 minutes; for a slightly more persistent taste 5/6 minutes are sufficient;
• pour into the cup gradually, tilting the teapot from time to time.

Here are some of the main varieties of green tea:

• *Bancha tea:*

it is the most common green tea. In Japan it is considered the everyday drink in fact Bancha means common tea.

• *Genmaicha tea:*

this type of tea is the union of Bancha tea with puffed rice and toasted rice. Its name means rice tea and can be easily used during meals due to its slightly salty taste.

• *Sencha tea:*

Sencha is a tea rich in vitamin A, antioxidant and antibacterial.

• *Hojicha tea:*

it is the tea that is obtained from the last harvest of Bancha and is considered to be the lowest quality of green tea because it is produced from the sticks and twigs of the plant rather than from the leaves. It is refreshing, has little caffeine, and is very light, lowers cholesterol, is antioxidant and antibacterial.

Macha tea:

Macha tea is made from Gyokuro. Among the Japanese green teas, Gyokuro is the most prized. It is harvested only once a year, between the end of April and the beginning of May, using the imperial method that captures only the terminal bud and, if the quality permits, the first leaf. The leaves are exposed to the sun for a long time in order to bring out the sweet taste of the plant. Its properties are many: it is rich in amino acids, vitamins and minerals; reduces cholesterol, helps fight flu symptoms.

Come e quando bere il tè verde durante la giornata:

A little trick used to encourage a sense of satiety and not suffer from a sense of hunger too, is to drink a glass of water about 30 minutes before the meal. Try replacing this glass of water with a cup of green tea before lunch for example. You will realize that it is an excellent remedy for calming hunger pangs.

You can apply this first trick every other day; on non-days, simply drink a large glass of natural water and you can drink a cup of green tea during lunch. Maybe you can choose Genmaicha tea, perfect with meals!

Drinking green tea during a meal can help not only keep your body hydrated but also promote the digestion process.

A cup of green tea between meals can be useful to replace those caloric snacks that sometimes you just can't help but create abdominal bloating. On the market you find mainly green tea in sachets but if you find time to go to the herbalist's shop or to a specialized shop you will find out how vast the reality of green tea is.

There are many ready-made drinks with green tea taste or made with green tea though

they do not have the same effects as a homemade cup of tea with real original and natural green tea leaves without the addition of chemicals or sugars.

I assure you that the taste is different too, if you get used to drinking the green tea made by you when you try to drink the green tea you buy at the supermarket, maybe contained in a plastic bottle, it will seem like you are drinking marsh water!

China is a large producer of green tea, some types of green tea produced in China are not widespread; the most delicate and sought after varieties, however, are Japanese green teas.

My advice is to verify that the purchased green tea is of natural, organic production and that it originates from controlled crops.

Chapter 5
Here's How To Gradually Eliminate Breakfast

"Breakfast of champions are not cereals, they are challenges."

(Nick Seitz)

Here is how you need to eliminate breakfast:

Week 1

- just wake up drink a glass of water

- after half an hour you have breakfast, reducing it by 10-15% and drinking green tea with a small teaspoon of honey and a little lemon

- during the morning, two hours after breakfast, drink water

Week 2

- just wake up drink a glass of water

- after half an hour you have breakfast, reducing it by 30% and drinking green tea with a very small teaspoon of honey and a little lemon

- during the morning, two hours after breakfast, drink water

Week 3

- just wake up drink a glass of water

- after half an hour you have breakfast, reducing it by 50% and drinking green tea without honey but only with a little lemon

- during the morning, two hours after breakfast, drink water

Week 4

- just wake up drink a glass of water

- after half an hour you have breakfast, reducing it by 75% and drinking green tea with lemon

- during the morning, two hours after breakfast, drink water

Week 5

- just wake up drink a glass of water

-after half an hour you have breakfast drinking only green tea with a little lemon

- during the morning, drink water

Let's take a practical example:

Week 1

Let's imagine that your breakfast consists of a cup of milk or coffee and 10 biscuits ...

What you will have to do in this first week is to eliminate milk or coffee and replace it with green tea, while for biscuits if you used to eat 10 of them this week you will eat 8 of them.

Week 2

In this second week you will simply have to eat 7 cookies and continue drinking green tea.

Week 3

In this third week you will simply have to eat 5 cookies and continue drinking green tea.

Week 4

In this fourth week you will simply have to eat 2 biscuits and continue drinking green tea.

Week 5

In this fifth week you will simply have to have breakfast only with green tea.

You will see that it will not be so difficult to get used to this new style of nutrition, but you will see that after a few weeks you will be completely used to it, you will end up with a lean, toned and healthy physique!

Follow everything literally, but above all do not leave this information in the form of a reading, put it into practice, otherwise this method will remain only one of the many methods read and never put into practice.

So what are you waiting for? Move!

Chapter 6
Find out how to further enhance the effects of this diet with the help of Ginger!

"If you really want to do something, you will find a way ... If you don't really want to, you will find an excuse."

(Jim Rohn)

But it does not end here ...

Here's how to further enhance the effects of this diet with the help of Ginger!

Perhaps not everyone knows that ginger, also called ginger and known by most as a valuable food flavoring, is also a root with slimming powers:

• **warms the body**

• **increases the temperature and perspiration**

• **helps eliminate excess fat and water**

Protagonist in the kitchen of original dishes and drinks, from centrifuged soups to desserts, this spice is a real concentrate of slimming properties, often unknown or underutilized. In this chapter I will explain in detail why ginger is effective for losing weight and in what concrete ways it is possible to exploit these virtues.

In fact, some research claims that this spice would be able to reduce the stimulation of hunger, thus promoting a more contained and reduced calorie intake. In addition, ginger warms the body which in turn speeds up the metabolism, in favor of a valid fat-melting action. The consumption of ginger allows you to burn calories faster as it promotes the digestion of carbohydrates and proteins. In addition, it helps the elimination of toxins and intestinal gas.

An interesting feature of this spice is its ability to burn calories, in fact ginger is part of the family of so-called thermogenic foods, that is, those that, in order to be assimilated, require a large expenditure of energy by the body. The hot and spicy flavor of this spice has the power to raise the body's temperature with an immediate effect on the acceleration of the basal metabolism.

Among the great properties of ginger for weight loss, the hypoglycemic one also stands out. In fact, this spice, by purifying the blood, is able to reduce the absorption of sugars, thus keeping blood sugar levels under control. This allows you to avoid the so-called glycemic peaks, the cause of a greater production of insulin, the hormone which, by signaling the presence of an excess of sugars in the brain, causes a slowing down of the metabolism and the formation of fat stores, especially at the abdominal level.

So taking this spice regularly helps to conquer or maintain a flat stomach. Among other things, ginger is also effective in case of swollen abdomen due to intestinal gas and excess yeast in the diet.

Reduce fluid buildup

Weight loss is not just about dissolving fatty deposits. If the goal is the remodeling of the body, it is also necessary to consider the stagnation of liquids that are concentrated in some typical areas (such as legs and buttocks) worsened by poor circulation. You must also take into account the digestive problems that cause abdominal bloating and also the slow metabolism that does not allow you to correctly transform food into energy. A truly effective slimming diet must consider all these aspects and, in this sense, ginger, acting on several fronts, is ideal to help you reach your weight goal. In fact, this spice counteracts abdominal swelling, stimulates diuresis and, as we have said, a detoxifying function for the body, as well as burning fat.

But where does ginger come from?

Ginger or rather the root of Zingiber officinalis, is a plant belonging to the Zingiberacee family (which includes 800 species).

The plant that develops from the tuberous root that we use and know as a spice can be approximately one meter tall. It is a perennial herb. The leaves and rhizomes have a fragrant smell when cut. They are white or yellow on the outside and become gray-brown or orange when they age and grow beyond 2.5 cm in diameter. This plant is believed to have originated in India and was later introduced to China.

Ginger has begun to make its appearance in food as a spice and in the world of folk medicine. Today it is mainly produced in

India, China and Thailand, although the Indian one remains of superior quality.

How to buy it?

If you decide to consume fresh ginger it is important to check that the zest is firm and compact, not wrinkled and without traces of mold. The rhizome must be full and, once cut, not too fibrous. The color must go, however, from white to yellow. Some more valuable species have bluish circles around the root. It is good to make sure that the ginger has been cultivated with organic cultivation methods and not treated with chemicals, above all we intend to use it for slimming or therapeutic purposes.

Remember to eliminate the stained parts at the time of use, with the help of a potato peeler to peel it. The root can be kept for a few weeks, after having wrapped it in greaseproof paper, in a closed glass jar and placed in the fridge. The powdered one, on the other hand, should be kept in a dry place away from light and consumed within a few weeks, before the active ingredients are dispersed or reduced.

Ginger also reduces inflammation.

University of Michigan scholars have found that ginger reduces colon inflammation and the risk of cancer. The subjects who had taken 2 grams per day of powdered ginger root for 4 weeks had a less inflamed intestine and more free from dangerous substances, the same that can favor the onset of tumors.

A study by the University of Kyoto and Ulsan highlights the effective action of ginger against chronic inflammatory states related to overweight, showing how this spice indirectly favors weight loss. In fact, excess fat triggers an inflammatory process that tends to become chronic and extend to the whole body. The body loses its ability to regulate itself, the percentage of fat increases and, consequently, also inflammation, triggering a real vicious circle.

For this reason, even if you are on a diet, if you are very overweight, it is often difficult to lose weight. Ginger helps inhibit the release of inflammatory substances into the blood, thus reducing the level of general inflammation and restoring normal hormonal functions that also regulate weight.

But how can ginger be used to lose weight? What are the best fat burning remedies based on this root and how to take them every day?

Now let's see together how to transform the most famous oriental spice into a weight loss ally, indicating a series of practical preparations that have different purposes: to purify, alleviate hunger, deflate, activate metabolism, etc.

The remedies that I will present are all simple to implement but highly effective.

First remedy: Purification

To be able to lose weight, the first step is to keep your body well cleansed by reducing the accumulation of pollutants and facilitating the natural expulsion of waste and toxins, too often accumulated.

To do this we can take advantage of the purifying qualities of ginger combined with green tea: these two foods together form a powerful "Detox" pair.

Blend 50 grams of green tea with 25 grams of dried ginger and 20 grams of mint leaves.

Leave to infuse for 8-10 minutes, filter and drink.

You can also take this drink throughout the morning during the morning fast.

Another useful remedy to detoxify the body is a cabbage and ginger smoothie.

To prepare it, blend 5 cabbage leaves, half a centimeter of fresh ginger, 2 mint leaves and half a glass of natural mineral water.

Drink on waking on an empty stomach.

To promote sweating and detoxify the body, you can also add this spice to the hot water of the bath for a "detox" bath.

Do this: grate 3 centimeters of ginger root and pour it into the water, along with half a cup of grated lemon peel. This also stimulates circulation.

Second remedy: cure the liver

When the liver is fatigued, losing weight is more difficult. In a good weight loss program, particular attention must therefore be paid to the purification of the liver gland.

Drain the liver with flavored water.

Whenever you feel the liver heavy, you can dilute the toxins present in the body by increasing the amount of liquids. To facilitate liver drainage it is therefore necessary to drink plenty of water (2 to 3 liters), preferably between meals: liquids help the body to expel toxins and waste.

If you struggle to drink smooth water, you can flavor it with a spoonful of lemon juice and a spoonful of ginger juice, mixing well.

Third remedy: improve digestion

Now let's see how to promote digestion and avoid abdominal bloating after meals. Sometimes even difficult digestion causes overweight. Just before going to sleep, to promote digestion and give you a good sleep, you can drink a warm infusion which, thanks to the beneficial properties of the herbs contained, gently stimulates the natural digestive process, also eliminating the abdominal swellings that often occur after a heavy or very high fiber meal.

Infuse for about 5-10 minutes, in a cup of boiling water, a generous spoonful of a mixture of the following herbs: mint, sage, fennel, cumin and ginger roots (you can also get the mix prepared by the herbalist).

Leave to cool for a few minutes, filter the liquid well and drink before going to sleep, without sweetening, if the infusion is too bitter and you just can't drink it, add a small teaspoon of organic honey.

To quickly dispose of the swelling of digestion and obtain a flatter belly, also increasing the sense of well-being and lightness, combine ginger with coriander.

Boil in one liter of cold water for 10-15 minutes 20 grams of powdered ginger root, 30 grams of fennel seeds, 20 grams of coriander seeds, 20 grams of orange zest and 10 grams of grapefruit zest (both organic) dried and chopped.

Let stand 5 minutes, then filter, let cool and keep this drink in the refrigerator, to consume it during the day.

Fourth remedy: dissolve fats

Ginger has a strong warming effect, which raises the body's temperature and speeds up the metabolism, making you burn more calories. In addition, its assimilation requires a high expenditure of energy, with a truly remarkable fat burning effect.

Combined with other natural substances active on metabolic processes, this spice is an extraordinary ally for your line. Now let's see some practical advice to make the most of its slimming properties.

If you have a tendency to put on weight even if you eat little, if you experience a constant sense of fatigue and notice a certain intestinal slowdown, maybe your metabolism needs a boost. You can awaken it with a stimulating herbal tea.

Infuse a teaspoon of green tea with three slices of fresh ginger and a teaspoon of dried rosemary: let it sit for 10 minutes, then filter.

Eat this herbal tea mid-morning and mid-afternoon for two weeks. Tea antioxidants help burn calories and promote lipolytic activity, while rosemary, like ginger, warms and invigorates the body.

Here is another mix of fat burning spices:

Spices are very important to reactivate the metabolism, burn more fat and calories, and achieve a slimming effect. If you combine ginger with other substances that stimulate thermogenesis, you can create an excellent spicy and slimming blend, among other things, to flavor fish, meat or vegetables, instead of salt.

Put in a glass jar (previously sterilized) a teaspoon of powdered ginger, one of saffron, one of ground coriander seeds and finish with half a teaspoon of black pepper and a pinch of nutmeg, mixing well.

Fifth remedy: quench hunger

Ginger helps you eat less without too much effort: thanks to its "warming" action, this spice quickly satisfies hunger and maintains a sense of satiety for longer.

Some minerals contained in ginger, together with other substances that calm anxiety and stress, help to calm the sudden appetite, of nervous origin, removing the insane desire to eat that comes only from the head, without meeting a real need of the body.

Do you fancy sugars?

Instead of throwing yourself on food, try this spicy drink that lowers blood sugar:

the ideal is an orange juice diluted with half a glass of apple juice, a pinch of ginger powder and a pinch of chilli pepper.

It is warming, relieves hunger and burns fat. Alternatively, acai juice is also excellent, the fruit of life that comes from the Amazon. In herbal medicine and in organic food stores you will find this ready made drink: drink half a glass with a pinch of ginger when you get the obsessive thought of sweets. With this zero-calorie drink you fill the hole in the stomach and do not gain weight.

If you are looking for something to eat less during meals, then do so:

30 minutes before main meals, drink an infusion of karcade, flavored with a pinch of powdered ginger: this herbal tea is excellent for those on a diet because it fills the stomach and prevents excesses at the table.

And with this we have also concluded the chapter on ginger, now you just have to get to work to burn fat even with the help of this wonderful spice.

Chapter 7
Wellness Superfoods of the 16: 8 DIET for weight loss by eating

If you think you are alone, know that it is not so. The desire for food, for a certain type of food, is very difficult to combat this because certain foods stimulate the production of certain substances in the brain that create, regardless of your will, the desire to eat further. Eating certain foods generates a food addiction which is the main cause of many health problems including being overweight and in severe cases obesity.

I myself have experienced firsthand what it means to feel the unstoppable desire for food, so strong that it seems uncontrollable.

But there is a way out, there is a way to take control of the situation and no longer be addicted to food.

What is the food you can't, or think you can't, do without? For me it was the desserts. Especially after lunch and even more after dinner I felt the need for a biscuit, a slice of cake or in any case a dessert or a baked product. At first I tried to resist but the only consequence was frustration and dissatisfaction and obviously after four or five days I started eating sweets again after lunch and after dinner with bad consequences on the belly - which continued to swell - and on the my mood.

Since I care a lot about my body, my well being and my health, I knew that it wasn't going well. My goal was to find an innovative way to eat in order to nourish my body and give it the substances it needs to function at its best without giving up the taste and pleasure of eating. I am convinced that eating is one of the pleasures of life.

I decided to learn as much as possible about nutrition and nutrition, I studied books, articles, scientific research, everything I could find on it. The most important thing I have learned, which I believe anyone who wants a better fitness should do, is to radically change the very concept of nutrition.

I began to see nutrition as a form of love and respect for my body, a means of nourishing it and giving it the way to function at its best. I wanted to learn to listen to his physical needs and not just my emotional desires.

So I had to find an alternative to the dessert after the meal that was able to satisfy both my desire and the physical needs of my body. Giving up was not the solution and it never is, which is why most restrictive diets prove ineffective.

I asked myself: "what can I eat that satisfies my desire for dessert and at the same time brings a nutritional value to my body"? It is clear that I could only find the answer with adequate information about the foods and their properties. For example, I found out what are the beneficial effects of dark chocolate and dried fruit and I found alternative and more beneficial recipes than I used to that allow me to prepare tasty dishes and not to give up the pleasure of eating. In a nutshell recipes that allowed me to combine business with pleasure.

The changes must be made one step at a time, day after day. If you are looking for a more beneficial alternative solution all your habits will change; today you will replace the milk chocolate with the dark one, tomorrow you will replace the refined white flour with the almond flour for example, the day after tomorrow you will try to eat a plate of brown red rice rather than the refined white one (organic red brown rice is one of the cereals that mostly frees blood from excess fats). For breakfast, I will drink green tea instead of milk (for a flat and slender belly, milk products should be avoided as much as possible).

The solution for a healthier and fitter physique and for a flat and slender belly is not in the elimination but in the replacement of food. The results on your fitness and well-being will be the simple consequence of the choices you make day after day.

The reason why many are attracted to foods rich in saturated fats and sugars is that, having deficiencies in essential nutrients, the body feels the need for foods that give immediate satisfaction and a sense of fullness like sweet and fried foods that they give a feeling of immediate satisfaction.

Foods like these, rich in sugar, refined flour, fats and yeasts taken in excess can damage the intestinal bacterial flora. If the intestinal bacterial flora is compromised, the organism does not correctly assimilate the nutritional principles of the food, the consequence is a malfunction of the metabolism and the accumulation of fat in the abdominal area.

In fact, not everything it fills nourishes but once you are used to feeding your body with foods rich in nutritional properties and with high nutritional value you will realize that you no longer feel that uncontrolled need for foods rich in sugars and saturated fats because you don't you will have more nutritional deficiencies.

The beneficial foods, the foods that are used to nourish - in the truest sense of the word - your body and therefore to provide it with energy and substances to make all organs work better, must contain nutritional properties and certain substances such as vitamins and minerals. The human body is perfect and knows how to stay healthy but you have to support it and show it respect by choosing what is most beneficial. Consider that your body always does everything you ask of it and if you treat it well it can do it at its best, if instead you fill it with harmful and difficult to dispose of substances it will make much more effort.

The foods that we consider Superfood given the high nutritional and beneficial power are foods that should never be missing from a food program in the name of well-being and a healthy and fit body as they perform multiple functions including:

- *help regulate the metabolism and not to accumulate fat,*
- *lower cholesterol levels,*
- *help prevent cardiovascular disease and cancer,*
- *help to cleanse the body,*
- *facilitate digestion and are rich in antioxidants which play a fundamental role in fighting the free radicals responsible for aging.*

Super Foods for snacks

Açai Berries

Oats

Avocado

Red fruits (Blueberries, Raspberries)

Dried fruit (Walnuts, Almonds)

Kefir

Pomegranate

Yogurt (natural low-fat white)

Super Foods for lunch and dinner

Green foods do

Salmon

Buckwheat

Barley

Quinoa

Super Foods to flavor

Seaweed

Lemons and Lime

Weight loss - www.benessereesalute.eu - All rights reserved

Hot pepper

Ginger

Misleading Super Foods:

Green foods don't

Legumes (lentils - azuki beans)

Garlic

onions

Oil seeds (Chia, Flax, Hemp, Sunflower)

Super Foods for snacks

Açai Berries:

The Açai Berries, originating in the South American rainforest, are the fruit of the Açai palm. For years considered as a Superfood, Açai berries such as blueberries are among the most beneficial berries for health because they contain numerous nutrients including minerals and vitamins.

Açai berries are rich in antioxidants and therefore are able to protect cells and counteract aging caused by the action of free radicals.

Studies have shown that the pulp of Açai berries is a substance capable of reducing the harmful effects of fatty foods. Açai berries are ideal for those who need to dispose of the excess kilos accumulated on the belly as they facilitate the digestion and detoxification of the body, help burn fat quickly and reduce swelling.

A spoonful of these berries, if taken as a snack, reduce hunger between meals.

Oats:

The main characteristic of oat flakes is the high fiber content, in particular of Beta-Glucan, which makes this food particularly healthy. Many scientific studies have shown that oats are a highly beneficial energy source for the body which reduces the level of cholesterol and blood sugar. One of the advantages of consuming oats, especially if you want to dispose of excess pounds, is its high satiating power. Oats are a source of vegetable proteins and unsaturated fats (the beneficial ones), vitamins, minerals and antioxidants.

Eating oatmeal with no added sugar, thanks to its high fiber and protein content, allows you to feel full for longer.

I really like to prepare oatmeal to be enjoyed with cinnamon and a teaspoon of honey. It is very simple to prepare and you can also enjoy it as a snack: for each portion use 35 gr. of oat flakes and 170 ml of water, bring to a boil and cook for about 15 minutes until the oats are cooked and creamy. Pour into a cup and add the cinnamon or other spices to taste, a teaspoon of honey and wanting dried fruit or raisins.

Avocado:

Avocado contains extremely healthy beneficial fats and is a highly nutritious fruit for the body. Rich in vitamins and minerals including potassium, an essential mineral that many are lacking in. The fats contained in avocado, including oleic acid, are comparable to those of olive oil. The fibers contained in avocado make it an excellent food for weight loss.

The monounsaturated fats contained in avocado help to reduce the chronic inflammation that generates the increase in cholesterol. They also prevent blood sugar spikes that cause the storage of excess calories in the form of fat especially on the belly and hips. The properties of avocado are able to balance hormones and prevent excessive production of cortisol (the stress hormone) which is one of the causes of obesity.

You can use avocado in many different ways and you can pair it with other sweet and savory foods. You can mash it to get tasty mousses to eat instead of mayonnaise. It is excellent with salmon, tomatoes and black olives. You can cut it into cubes and add it to the salad.

The red fruits:

The fruit with dark red, blue and black shades has a high content of antioxidants with known protective effects on blood circulation and capillary fragility. Strawberries, for example, are an excellent source of potassium, fiber, vitamins B / C / K, magnesium and Omega-3.

Blueberries contain over 20 types of anthocyanins, i.e. antioxidants with a characteristic blue - violet color capable of counteracting various cell aging and tissue aging processes. Raspberries and blackberries contain many fibers; a cup of these fruits is able to provide you with 1/3 of the daily fiber requirement.

But why are these antioxidants so important?

The reason is that when a cell contains many free radicals, the so-called oxidative stress occurs which leads to the production of chemicals that promote the appearance of inflammation inside the cell. Antioxidants (flavonoids and vitamin E for example) counteract the action of free radicals.

Cranberries are natural probiotics or microorganisms that prove able, once ingested in adequate quantities, to perform beneficial functions for the organism in particular facilitate digestion and contribute to the health of the gastrointestinal tract.

To fully enjoy all the nutritional properties and the multiple beneficial effects of red fruits it is necessary to include them in adequate quantities in your food program. I suggest you give yourself a portion of red fruit once a day. You can consume red fruits as they are or add them to natural low-fat yogurt or kefir. You can eat them as a snack between meals.

Dried fruit:

Numerous studies confirm the beneficial effects of dried fruit, in particular walnuts and almonds represent an excellent food rich in Omega-3 and vitamin E with well-known antioxidant properties (property that counteracts aging).

Walnuts and almonds are very useful for keeping the blood cholesterol level and the risk of cardiovascular disease under control. Overweight and obesity are excellent allies of cardiovascular disease, all the more reason to include dried fruit in your food program. Furthermore, being rich in fiber, dried fruit is an excellent choice for a snack as it promotes a sense of satiety.

However, you must not exceed the quantities in fact almonds and in particular walnuts also have a high calorific value.

Abdominal fat not only affects the aesthetic aspect but is associated with serious health problems such as chronic inflammations and cardiovascular diseases. Monounsaturated fats make dried fruit an effective food for weight loss on the belly.

I eat them in every way, as a snack or in a salad.

Kefir

Have you ever heard of kefir? The origin of this word comes from Turkish and means "feeling good". It is a fermented milk drink with a characteristic pungent and sparkling taste.

Contains protein, calcium, phosphorus, vitamin B and magnesium.

Although it is a very ancient drink, it is not so widespread probably because its effects and beneficial properties are not fully known. Compared to yogurt which contains about 4% sugar, kefir only contains 1%.

Kefir is rich in nutrients and probiotics extremely beneficial for the health of the intestinal bacterial flora. The beneficial effects of kefir are evident especially with regard to the digestive system, weight control if combined with a balanced diet, and a general feeling of well-being and vitality of the body and mind. You can combine it with fresh fruit for a beneficial and nutritious snack. Some compare it to yogurt but in reality the beneficial effects on the intestinal bacterial flora of kefir are much higher and stronger than yogurt.

It is very easy and quick to prepare, but the first time it is necessary to obtain the grains from those who already produce it. Kefir grains are not sold in stores but can be found by those who love and care for this product by doing a brief search, even online, making sure that they are biologically controlled micro kefir grains.

You need a jar (preferably glass) and kefir grains. Add milk because the grains are live cultures and stay alive thanks to the milk lactose which they absorb and transform into a fermented drink. For the proportions generally 1 lt of milk is used per 100gr. of kefir granules.

Let it sit for about 24 hours before passing it in a colander. By passing it in the colander you will get a drink with a creamy consistency and in the colander you will always have new kefir grains ready to repeat the procedure and prepare more or even to share with your friends who want to try this concentrate of well-being.

Now I would like to give you some advice that will help you make your kefir even tastier and a little less pungent. You can use the zest of a lemon or an orange and actually almost any type of fruit and add it to your kefir and let it rest for the usual 24 hours.

Pomegranate:

Certainly recognized as one of the healthiest fruits in the world, pomegranate contains phytonutrients that cannot be found in other foods. Some of the substances that pomegranate contains are vitamins, minerals and fiber but above all bioactive plant compounds with countless beneficial properties for health.

Pomegranate contains a unique substance called punicalagina and is a very powerful antioxidant capable of reducing inflammation. Consuming pomegranate improves energy and helps to counteract tiredness.

Many studies agree that pomegranate has the power to significantly reduce abdominal fat. The substances contained in the pomegranate hinder the development of fat cells in the waistline. The juice contained within the pomegranate seeds reduces the level of unesterified fatty acids in the blood. A high level of non-esterified fatty acids can lead to increased fat storage in the abdomen.

You can eat the beans as they are in a cup with a teaspoon between meals. Pomegranate is very good with brown rice. In a saucepan add a cup of brown red rice with three cups of water and cook until the water has evaporated completely. When cooked, add saffron and serve on a plate. Add two or three tablespoons of pomegranate.

The Yogurt:

The beneficial properties of natural low-fat yogurt are given by the high nutritional value due to an excellent balance of calcium and proteins. The high degree of acidity of yogurt makes proteins more digestible than milk and facilitates their absorption.

During the preparation phase, lactose or the milk sugar present in yogurt is fermented, making it digestible even for those who are intolerant to milk.

The consumption of yogurt has the property of reducing the formation of hydrogen sulphide which is the cause of halitosis and colon cancer.

Another important aspect related to the intake of yogurt is the property that it has to strengthen the immune system against the activity of fungi, bacteria and viruses.

The B vitamins that are supplied by lactic ferments have a protective action against the liver and intestines; lactic acid instead has the property of promoting the absorption of calcium and phosphorus.

Natural low-fat yogurt is a food rich in vitamins, minerals and enzymes beneficial for our health.

Yogurt contains live microorganisms that allow this food to exert an anti-infective and antitoxic action useful for restoring the bacterial flora and stimulating intestinal activity.

Between one meal and another, pour the natural low-fat yogurt into a cup and consume it naturally or with the addition of a drop of honey, red fruits or dried fruit. It is also very good with sunflower seeds or raisins.

Super Foods for lunch and dinner

Green foods do:

The foods belonging to this group are: asparagus, basil, spinach, white grapes and courgettes.

These green foods contain chlorophyll and carotenoids and are therefore excellent antioxidants. These are elements that have a general beneficial effect on the tissues and help to maintain a youthful appearance by counteracting the action of free radicals that are the main ones responsible for aging.

Green foods promote iron absorption and are rich in minerals.

All green vegetables and vegetables help regulate the metabolism of fats and sugars, have a detoxifying action and the precious minerals with which these foods are rich contribute to strengthening bones, blood vessels, eyesight and teeth.

Asparagus

Asparagus acts as a diuretic to reduce water retention which causes abdominal bloating. Asparagus is an excellent source of inulin, a dietary fiber that keeps the digestive system healthy and decreases constipation and other stomach and intestinal tract disorders.

Basil

Basil fights aerophagia and meteorism. A herbal tea made from basil and fennel is an excellent remedy for heaviness and bloating.

Spinach

Spinach has few calories and countless beneficial properties. The high calcium content helps strengthen muscle structure and tone the abs.

White grapes

For the digestive system it is useful to eat white grapes without peel and without seeds.

Zucchini

Zucchini have few calories, many vitamins and minerals. The peel of the courgettes is rich in fiber which helps to reduce constipation.

You can use these foods not only as a side dish but also as a unique dish to pair with brown red rice, quinoa, or barley. As basic ingredients for soups or baked with spices. The basil instead gives more flavor to your dishes and thus help you to reduce the seasonings.

Salmon:

Salmon is very rich in Omega-3 which represent a category of essential fatty acids essential for the well-being of the organism. The presence of Omega-3 counteracts aging and some studies show that these fatty acids also play an antidepressant role. Omega-3s are useful in the prevention of some tumors and are adjuvants in the treatment of rheumatoid arthritis.

Salmon brings significant quantities of vitamin D which positively affects the absorption of calcium and promotes the mineralization of the skeleton.

Salmon is an excellent food rich in proteins, has many nutritional properties and increases the metabolism and also contributes to lowering the cholesterol level.

It is preferable to consume non-farmed salmon and specifically wild Alaskan red salmon, as it contains a higher amount of Omega-3 than the farmed one and has negligible quantities of pollutants as well as scarce traces of mercury.

Salmon provides a lot of energy, reduces chronic inflammation (the cause of being overweight), tones the muscle mass and increases the calorie burning process.

Salmon is very tasty and requires no seasoning except a pinch of Himalayan pink salt and freshly ground pepper. You can cook it in a non-stick pan or in the oven and consume it with a vegetable garnish. I eat salmon also raw (naturally it must be very fresh) in this case it is excellent with freshly ground black pepper and avocado mousse.

Buckwheat:

Buckwheat is so rich in beneficial properties that it is considered among the various foods that are part of the medicine foods. This food provides energy and vigor and its proteins have the highest biological value in the plant kingdom.

Buckwheat is rich in minerals and antioxidants. One of the great advantages of this food is its ability to regulate the blood sugar level. As we have seen previously, the spikes and drops in blood sugar represent one of the main causes of hunger attacks and mood swings. That's why it is important to choose foods that release sugars gradually, without creating imbalances.

Buckwheat is qualitatively superior to rice, wheat and corn, above all because it has a lower glycemic index and is more protein. Buckwheat does not contain gluten and does not generate abdominal swelling.

Buckwheat can be consumed as a cereal or buckwheat flour can be used as a more nutritious and beneficial alternative to refined white flour.

Barley:

Beta-Glucan, a natural element of plant origin present in barley, lowers blood glucose levels and reduces LDL cholesterol (the harmful one).

There are different types of barley on the market including, for example, hulled barley and pearl barley. These two types undergo refining processes that cause the loss of many nutrients in the food such as fiber, vitamins and mineral salts. Make sure you always buy whole barley and possibly organic barley, to fully preserve all the typical properties of this precious cereal.

Barley is a cereal with a soft consistency similar to pasta and is an excellent source of minerals and fibers that promote intestinal regularity. Barley promotes weight loss as it has a high satiating power with few calories but countless nutrients.

You can add barley to your soups or given its rich and intense flavor, similar to hazelnuts, you can choose it as an ingredient for snacks to alternate with oat flakes. I like it very much cooked as a risotto, with vegetables and saffron or with leeks, pine nuts and raisins.

Quinoa

Quinoa has also recently become popular in our kitchens but is actually a very ancient food, originally from Peru, and was the basis of the Inca people 's diet. Considered a food of the gods, Quinoa does not contain gluten, it is not wheat but a protein food in reality they are the seeds of a herbaceous plant. Given the innumerable beneficial properties (very rich source of fiber and minerals), Quinoa is considered a Superfood and is very good.

To eliminate swelling and excess fat, foods such as quinoa are indicated: rich in fiber and protein that help the metabolism to burn fat and have a gradual release of energy that prevents drops in sugar and therefore attacks of hunger sudden.

We recommend rinsing Quinoa before cooking to eliminate saponin which is a slightly bitter substance present in this plant.

It is very simple to prepare: boil two cups of water for each cup of Quinoa, when the water boils pour the Quinoa with a pinch of salt and cook until all the water has evaporated.

Once the Quinoa is cooked you can sauté it in the pan with vegetables such as carrots and courgettes, you can add chopped chicken for a delicious single dish and even want some olives. Otherwise you can incorporate it to soups.

Super Foods to flavor

Algae:

There are different types of seaweed on the market including: Nori, Dulse, Kombu, Kelp, Arame, Irish Moss, Alaria Esculenta. You can buy seaweed in organic stores and in many supermarkets in the bio / vegan department.

Seaweed contains minerals, a wide range of vitamins and valuable antioxidants to combat cellular aging. But the real precious and practically unavailable element in other more common foods is iodine

Obesity, the accumulation of fat, is one of the consequences of an inflammatory state of the metabolic tissues within the body. Sea algae counteract the body's chronic inflammation caused by the accumulation of fat;

In Japan, seaweed is a fundamental food and can be found in Miso soup as well as in Sushi and other typical Japanese dishes.

For example, Nori seaweed is a sheet of pasta in which you can put vegetables, quinoa, avocado and salmon to create delicious rolls.

The seaweed of Brittany is also very good and occurs in dried flakes to be rehydrated in cold water for a few minutes. They can be used as an aromatic herb, cooked or raw to flavor dishes.

Lemons and Lime:

Like most citrus fruits, lemons and limes are also divided into 8/10 segments, each segment is a concentrate of beneficial properties including flavonoid compounds with antioxidant properties. Lemons and limes are rich in phytonutrients and vitamin C essential for the well-being of cells. The vitamin C contained in lemons is able to increase the absorption of iron, this is one of the reasons why it is recommended to add lemon juice to the steaks.

A decoction of sage and lemon or lime promotes digestion. Lemon and lime help strengthen the immune system and reduce swelling.

I really use all of both lemons and limes, in fact I buy them fresh and freeze them so that they are always ready to be grated on numerous dishes. Half a lemon juice in a glass of warm water is the best way to do an internal cleansing of the body. The zest of the lemon gives flavor to yogurt, fish, vegetables, brown red rice, chicken. You can really use it at will on almost any dish.

Hot pepper:

Spicy chilli is a thermogenic food with multiple organoleptic properties.

The characteristic characteristic of thermogenic foods is their ability to increase metabolism and burn more calories thanks to thermogenesis, a metabolic process which consists in the production of heat by the body mainly in the adipose tissue

Chili pepper dissolves blood clots and therefore stimulates blood circulation and protects capillaries. Some chilli compounds, including flavonoids, have an antibacterial effect.

The hot pepper is rich in vitamin C and has a strong antioxidant power, promotes intestinal functions, prevents fermentation and the formation of intestinal gas and toxins.

The capsaicin contained in the pepper makes it a thermogenic food that increases the consumption of calories and promotes weight loss.

Use chili pepper to give more flavor to your vegetable dishes, to flavor chicken meat and soups. I always recommend not to abound because little chilli enhances the flavor of the dishes while an excessive dose burns the palate and the flavors are no longer felt.

Misleading Super Foods

I have called these foods "deceptive" because although they are known to be considered very healthy and are rich in beneficial and nutritional properties, they are not suitable for weight loss. While some foods promote the melting of fats others ferment and create abdominal bloating.

Among these foods that cause abdominal bloating, constipation and in some cases even cramps in the abdomen, there are FODMAPs (Fermentable, Oligo saccharides, Disaccharides, Monosaccharides and Polyols). These are short chain carbohydrates which can generate digestive disorders.

Among the foods - considered superfoods - but which have a high FODMAP content and are therefore contraindicated for weight loss we find:

Green foods don't:

The foods belonging to this group are: artichokes, broccoli, cabbage.

As with green foods, yes, these green foods also contain chlorophyll and are therefore excellent antioxidants. They have a general beneficial effect on the tissues and help to maintain a youthful appearance by counteracting the action of free radicals that are the main ones responsible for aging.

Green foods promote iron absorption and are rich in minerals.

All green vegetables and vegetables help regulate the metabolism of fats and sugars, have a detoxifying action and the precious minerals with which these foods are rich contribute to strengthening bones, blood vessels, eyesight and teeth.

Not only as a side dish but also as a unique dish to combine with brown red rice, quinoa, or barley. As basic ingredients for soups or baked with spices. Basil and parsley, on the other hand, can give more flavor to your dishes and thus help you reduce seasonings.

Although green foods such as artichokes, broccoli and cabbage are considered superfoods with innumerable beneficial properties, they are not suitable for a weight loss diet.

Beans and lentils - azuki beans:

Beans and lentils, but legumes in general, are rich in vegetable proteins, have an important amount of vitamins and fiber and help accelerate intestinal transit by promoting detoxification.

Legumes represent a valid energy source thanks to their carbohydrate content; they are the main source of protein after food of animal origin and the few fats contained are mainly unsaturated (the beneficial ones). In addition, legumes are particularly rich in fiber, useful in the control of sugars and cholesterol in the blood. It is a food with very high nutritional properties thanks also to the content of minerals such as phosphorus, potassium, calcium and iron.

Beans are the most fiber-rich legumes while lentils are particularly energetic due to their rich starch content. Lentils have a fair iron content and have the advantage of being among the fastest-cooking legumes.

In Japan it is the most consumed legume after soy, it is Azuki beans. Azuki beans are small and dark red in color with excellent nutritional properties.

This food is sometimes improperly called red soybean because of its color. Azuki contain minerals and trace elements such as potassium, zinc, molybdenum and iron. Azuki beans are naturally rich in B vitamins, contain fiber and protein. In addition, these legumes help the formation of enzymes useful to the liver and have purifying and diuretic properties.

These beans are easily digestible, low in fat and also contain isoflavones, substances that can keep our immune system, brain and bones healthy.

In typical oriental cuisine, Azuki beans are ground and boiled to form a puree to which raw cane sugar is added to make it a sweet-tasting cream. Azuki beans, like most legumes, must be left to soak before being consumed. I suggest you not to throw away the water when you drain them but to drink it as it is rich in minerals and vitamins very useful for your body.

You can eat legumes, and especially beans, both cooked as a single dish and cold in a salad. They are excellent with a thinly cut fresh spring onion.

Although legumes are considered superfoods with innumerable beneficial properties, they are not indicated in a weight loss diet.

Garlic:

Garlic is a natural antibacterial able to strengthen the immune system and reduce cholesterol. Garlic has an extraordinary purifying power and the ability to fight hypertension. Thanks to the high content of phosphorus and sulfur it has a calming effect on the nervous system.

To fully enjoy all the countless beneficial effects of this food, you should consume it raw.

Garlic is a Super Food used since ancient times as a natural medicine. The beneficial power of garlic is given by the enormous amount of minerals it contains in addition to vitamins, in particular vitamins of group C and group B. A clove of garlic, if used raw to flavor, is a natural antibiotic.

You can mash it and use it to season vegetables, add it to soups, prepare excellent sauces such as Guacamole (avocado-based), hummus (chickpea-based) or Tapenade (olive-based).

Although garlic is considered a superfood with innumerable beneficial properties, it is not indicated in a weight loss diet.

Onion:

Onions are excellent antioxidants for our body and contain numerous mineral salts and trace elements. Onions are rich in iron, magnesium, potassium and phosphorus, they are also rich in vitamins and constitute a natural antibacterial able to stimulate the immune system.

Onions stimulate diuresis, rebalance the intestinal bacterial flora and help to lower blood sugar levels.

To keep its properties unaltered, it is preferable to consume it raw or steamed.

Onion is really a versatile ingredient to use to flavor many dishes, from leafy salads to legumes. You can cook them in the oven stuffed with other vegetables. You can prepare a tuna and onion appetizer or use them as a base for tasty vegetable creams.

Although onion is considered a superfood with countless beneficial properties, it is not suitable for a weight loss diet.

Oil seeds:

(Chia, Flax, Hemp, Sunflower)

Seeds are the embryos of plants and represent the very origin of nutrition. Oil seeds are a concentrate of vitamins, minerals, essential oils and beneficial enzymes for the body. Chia seeds and hemp seeds are an excellent source of Omega3 fatty acids and alpha linoleic acid, flax seeds are rich in fiber. Sunflower seeds are a concentrate of vitamin E, the most important antioxidant for the body.

To assimilate all the beneficial effects, the seeds must always be chewed and eaten raw without adding salt or sugars. Use oilseeds to crunch salad, add them to yogurt or oatmeal. If you leave a teaspoon of chia seeds in half a glass of water, a gelatinous substance will form which many use as a substitute for eggs to prepare different recipes or you can drink this same compound for a concentrate of well-being given by these precious seeds.

Although oilseeds are considered superfoods with innumerable beneficial properties, they are not indicated in a weight loss diet.

The first fruits of the season

Choose Superfoods and combine them with the first fruits of the season for greater freshness and quality, each season has its Wellness and Beauty Elixir.

Mother Nature offers you real concentrates of wellness and beauty, which you can bring to your table. When you go shopping, keep these tips in mind below and stock up on these nutrient-dense foods. When you buy fruit and vegetables you always prefer fresh and seasonal ones and if possible buy organic products, of controlled origin and from your trusted greengrocer

Elixir of Wellness and Autumn Beauty

Vegetables:

Pumpkin - Cabbage - Cabbage Broccoli - Savoy Cabbage - Cauliflower - Broccoli - Turnip tops - Brussels sprouts - Celery - Leeks - Spring onions - Garlic - Onions.

Fruits:

Pomegranate - Grapes - Dried Fruit - Apples - Oranges - Tangerines - Grapefruits - Cedars - Pears - Figs - Persimmon.

Elixir of Wellness and Winter Beauty

Vegetables:

Pumpkin - Artichokes - Asparagus - Radishes - Cabbage - Cabbage Broccoli - Savoy Cabbage - Cauliflower - Broccoli -

Aubergines - Turnip tops - Brussels sprouts - Celery - Thistles - Leeks - Leeks - Spring onions - Garlic - Onions.

Fruits:

Kiwi - Mandarins - Grapefruits - Oranges - Cedars - Pears - Apples.

Elixir of Wellness and Spring Beauty

Vegetables:

Artichokes - Courgettes - Asparagus - Tomatoes - Spring onions - Radishes - Aubergines - Broad beans - Peas - Green beans - Snow peas - Garlic - Shallots - Onions.

Fruits:

Strawberries - Cherries - Apricots - Melons.

Elixir of Wellness and Summer Beauty

Vegetables:

Peppers - Tomatoes - New Potatoes - Zucchini - Leeks - Spring Onions - Green Beans - Broad Beans - Peas.

Fruits:

Berries - Watermelon - Melons - Apricots - Peaches - Strawberries - Plums - Plums.

Chapter 8
70 yummy recipes 16: 8 KETO DIET burns fat

If you really want to push and increase your metabolism to burn more fat, then you should consider adding keto meals (especially at dinner) to the 16: 8 DIET.

Tons of celebrities are jumping on the 16: 8 Keto DIET bandwagon, and for good reason. The two systems work hand in hand to accelerate weight loss, not to mention many other health benefits. Fasting combined with keto meals is an extraordinary tool for improving your biology. It's free. It is universally accessible. It is adaptable.

Here are some of its benefits:

Double the fat loss

Eating all meals in an 8-hour window (for example, eating between noon and 8:00 pm and fasting the other 16 hours a day) causes significant weight loss without counting calories. While this type of intermittent fasting causes weight loss regardless of what people eat, research shows that people who do it healthily lose twice the weight (7% versus 3% of their body weight) than those who fast while continuing to eat junk. So it is even more important to follow a high-performance diet such as the ketogenic diet.

Makes the skin elastic

GH naturally drops with age. But when subjects were given GH supplements, not only did they lose fat and build muscle, but their skin thickness also improved, making it stronger and more resistant to sagging and wrinkles.

Intermittent fasting and the ketogenic diet together bring GH to the stars!

Slows down aging

Fasting increases the production of stem cells. Stem cells are like organic pasta - your body transforms them into any type of cell it needs and uses them to replace old or damaged cells, keeping you younger at the cellular level. Stem cells are perfect for the skin, joints, old lesions, chronic pains and more. You can try stem cell therapy ... or you can simply fast.

Improve brain function

Fasting also helps build a better brain. Intermittent fasting increases a protein in the brain called BDNF that researchers have nicknamed "Miracle for your brain." BDNF improves learning and memory and can help you forge stronger neuronal pathways, making your brain faster and more efficient is especially important when you get older.

Stimulates autophagy

Autophagy is spring cleansing for your cells. Autophagy means "self-eating", which is spot on: when the autophagy turns on, your cells sift through their internal parts, eliminate everything that is damaged or old and install new bright versions. Autophagy is like a tuning for your car: it flows more fluid after all. It reduces inflammation and also increases longevity. Intermittent fasting triggers, to quote the researchers, "profound" autophagy, especially in the brain.

Lowers inflammation

Intermittent fasting reduces oxidative stress and inflammation markers at the body level. Inflammation is one of the major factors of poor performance, aging and disease. Keeping inflammation low will increase your longevity and help your body function better.

In short, intermittent fasting is like a broad spectrum update for your body. The fact that your biology responds to fasting by becoming stronger makes sense from an evolutionary point of view: it is precisely when you are short of food that you have to run your best, to increase your chances of finding something to eat to survive.

The only problem with intermittent fasting

There is one main disadvantage of intermittent fasting: it is possible to have unstable blood sugar if you are eating a lot of carbohydrates.

If you experience intermittent fasting on a higher carbohydrate diet, your blood sugar will rise and fall significantly during the day. It will be higher after the meal, then gradually decrease as you go into your fast. Unstable blood sugar brings additional challenges to fasting:

Lack of energy.

When you have nothing in the system for several hours, your blood sugar level will drop at the end of the reporting period. If you've ever had a blood sugar problem, you know how it feels in this state. Drowsiness, concentration problems, dizziness, intense cravings and occasional mood swings generally accompany a low blood sugar level. Your cells are running out of fuel and start asking to give them more carbohydrates.

You will spike blood sugar when you eat.

If you are fasting on a high carbohydrate diet and have fed the cravings and lack of energy from low blood sugar levels, there is a good chance that you will eat a lot of carbohydrates in your meal. You want to eat large meals when you fast to make sure you have enough calories, but all those excess carbohydrates in one fell swoop will increase your blood sugar in the opposite direction, from bottom to top. Hyperglycaemia causes fatigue and lack of concentration. That violent hunger will also make you binge unnecessarily, and any carbohydrate you don't use will be stored as fat.

If your blood sugar level goes up and down all day, you will never feel stable and reliable energy, which will make fasting quite difficult. ***This is where the ketogenic diet comes in.***

Why does the ketogenic diet and intermittent fasting accelerate weight loss?

With a ketogenic diet, you stop eating carbohydrates and replace them with foods rich in protein and fat. After a few days of taking a few carbohydrates, your body becomes efficient at burning fat for fuel. You walk in fat-burning mode all day, enjoying some exclusive benefits:

• **No desire.** Fat does not increase blood sugar levels. In fact, a keto diet is so effective at stabilizing blood sugar that it completely excluded type II diabetics, according to a recent study. If you combine a keto diet with fasting, your blood sugar level will remain stable and low (but not too low) throughout the day. Say goodbye to cravings, tiredness and mood swings that make fasting with carbohydrates so difficult.

• **Suppression of hunger.** A ketogenic diet also suppresses hunger. With a ketogenic diet, your liver transforms fat into small bundles of energy called ketones, which it then sends through the bloodstream for your cells to be used as fuel. Ketones suppress ghrelin, your body's main hunger hormone. The high ghrelin makes you hungry. With the ketogenic diet, your ghrelin remains low, even when you have no food in your system. In other words, you can go longer without eating and you won't be hungry. Fasting becomes significantly easier with the ketogenic diet, so you can fast for longer windows to take advantage of all the benefits.

• **Fat loss.** The ketogenic diet and intermittent fasting are a very powerful mix for losing weight. Fasting and the ketogenic diet spontaneously increase fat loss, even when people do not intentionally limit their calories. When you pair intermittent fasting with the ketogenic diet together, you become a fat burning machine. Weight drops rapidly, and since keto also suppresses ghrelin, you never experience the feeling of hunger and sadness from the deprivation that usually accompany weight loss.

Intermittent fasting and the ketogenic diet are the perfect couple to lose weight quickly!

Seeing is believing…

TABLE OF CONTENTS Recipes 16:8 KETO DIET

LUNCH RECIPES
SOUP RECIPES
KETO BROCCOLI SOUP
KETO TACO SOUP
KETO CHICKEN SOUP
KETO SPINACH SOUP
KETO TOSCANA SOUP
KETO PARMESAN SOUP
KETO CAULIFLOWER SOUP
KETO BROCCOLI CHEESE SOUP
KETO QUESO SOUP
KETO CRAB SOUP
SALAD
KETO SALAD
KETO BROCCOLI SALAD
KETO GREEN SPRING SALAD
KETO EGG SALAD
KETO CAESAR SALAD
KETO PEPPERONI SALAD
KETO CHICKEN SALAD
KETO TUNA SALAD
SPINACH SALAD
KETO POTOTO SALAD

DINNER RECIPES
KETO MONGOLAIN BEEF
PEPPERONI KETO PIZZA
QUICK KETO PIZZA
MUSHROOMS PIZZA
BUFFALO KETO CHICKEN TENDERS
KETO LASAGNA
KETO PARMESAN CASSEROLE
KETO CHEESE MEATBALLS

KETO CHEESY BACON CHICKEN
KETO CHEESEBURGER

DESSERT RECIPES
CAKE
CHEESECAKE KETO FAT BOMBS
KETO BROWNIES
KETO ICE CREAM
KETO EGG CREPES
KETO NAAN
PEANUT BUTTER COOKIES
BUTTERY KETO CREPES
KETO LEMON FAT BOMB
PEANUT BUTTER BALLS
NUT FREE KETO BROWNIE
SMOOTIES
COFFEE SMOOTHIE
CHAI PUMPKIN SMOOTHIE
CASHEW SMOOTHIE
BREAKFAST SMOOTHIE
KETO MILKSHAKE SMOOTHIE
AVOCADO SMOOTHIE
COLLAGEN SMOOTHIE
FAT BOMB SMOOTHIE
CINNAMON SMOOTHIE
TROPICAL SMOOTHIE

LUNCH RECIPES
(SOUP RECIPES)

KETO BROCCOLI SOUP

Serves: 4
Prep Time: 10   Minutes
Cook Time: 30   Minutes
Total Time: 40   Minutes

INGREDIENTS

- olive oil
- 1 cup chicken broth
- 1 cup heavy whipping cream
- 6 oz. shredded cheddar cheese
- salt
- 5-ounces broccoli
- 1 celery stalk
- 1 small carrot
- ½ onion

DIRECTIONS

1. In a pot add olive oil over medium heat

2. Add onion, carrot, celery and cook for 2-3 minutes

3. Add chicken broth and simmer for 4-5 minutes

4. Stir in broccoli and cream

5. Sprinkle in cheese and season with salt

KETO TACO SOUP

Serves: 8
Prep Time: 10 Minutes
Cook Time: 10 Minutes
Total Time: 20 Minutes

INGREDIENTS

- 2 lbs. ground beef
- 1 onion
- 1 cup heavy whipping cream
- 1 tsp chili powder
- 14 oz. cream cheese
- 1 tsp garlic
- 1 tsp cumin
- 2 10 oz. cans tomatoes
- 16 oz. beef broth

DIRECTIONS

1. Cook for a couple of minutes, onion, garlic and beef

2. Add cream cheese and stir until fully melted

3. Add tomatoes, whipping cream, beef broth, stir and bring to boil

KETO CHICKEN SOUP

Serves:4
Prep Time: 10   Minutes
Cook Time: 30   Minutes
Total Time: 40   Minutes

INGREDIENTS

- 2 boneless chicken breast
- 20-ounces diced tomatoes
- ½ tsp salt
- 1 cup salsa
- 6-ounces cream cheese
- avocado
- 2 tablespoons taco seasoning
- 1 cup chicken broth

DIRECTIONS

1. In a slow cooker place all ingredients and cook for 5-6 hours or until chicken is tender

2. Whisk cream cheese into the broth

3. When ready, remove and serve

KETO SPINACH SOUP

Serves: 2
Prep Time: 5   Minutes
Cook Time: 15   Minutes
Total Time: 20   Minutes

INGREDIENTS

- ¼ lbs. spinach
- 2 oz. onion
- ¼ lbs. heavy cream
- ½ oz. garlic
- 1 chicken stock cube
- 1,5 cup water
- 1 tablespoons butter

DIRECTIONS

1. In a saucepan melt the butter and sauté the onion

2. Add garlic, spinach and stock cube and half the water

3. Cook until spinach wilts

4. Pour everything in a blender and blend, add water

5. Serve with pepper and toasted nuts

KETO TOSCANA SOUP

Serves: 4
Prep Time: 10   Minutes
Cook Time: 30   Minutes
Total Time: 40   Minutes

INGREDIENTS

- 1 lb. Italian sausage
- ½ cup whipping cream
- 1 tsp garlic
- 2 cup kale leaves
- 1 bag radishes 16-ounces
- 1 onion
- 30-ounces vegetable broth

DIRECTIONS

1. Cut radishes into small chunks and blend until smooth

2. In a pot add onion and sausage, cook until brown, add radishes, broth

3. Cook on medium heat, add heavy whipping cream, kale leaves

4. Cook for a couple minutes

5. Remove and serve

KETO PARMESAN SOUP

Serves:4
Prep Time: 10 Minutes
Cook Time: 30 Minutes
Total Time: 40 Minutes

INGREDIENTS

- 1 broccoli
- 1 tsp pepper
- 1 tablespoon butter
- 1 tablespoon cheese
- 1 onion
- ½ cup warm
- 1 tsp salt
- ½ cup heavy cream

DIRECTIONS

1. In a saucepan add onion and cook

2. Stir in broccoli and cook until soft

3. Combine with heavy cream and place in a blender, blend until smooth

4. Return the soup to the saucepan, season with salt

5. Serve and sprinkle with parmesan

KETO CAULIFLOWER SOUP

Serves:4
Prep Time: 10   Minutes
Cook Time: 30   Minutes
Total Time: 40   Minutes

INGREDIENTS

- ½ head of cauliflower
- ½ cup heavy cream
- ½ red bell pepper
- 1 tsp salt
- 1 tsp pepper
- 1 tablespoon butter
- 1 tablespoons parmesan cheese
- 1 tsp herbs

DIRECTIONS

1. In a saucepan melt butter, add cauliflower and cook until soft

2. Remove from saucepan and set aside

3. Melt butter and sauté and bell pepper

4. In a food processor add cauliflower mixture, pepper and cook for 4-5 minutes

5. Season with salt and pepper

6. Garnish with parmesan and serve

KETO BROCCOLI CHEESE SOUP

Serves: 2
Prep Time: 10   Minutes
Cook Time: 20   Minutes
Total Time: 30   Minutes

INGREDIENTS

- 2 cups broccoli
- 3 cups chicken broth
- 1 onion
- 1 cup heavy cream
- 6 oz. cream cheese
- 1 tablespoon hot sauce
- 3 tablespoons butter
- 1 clove garlic
- 6 oz. cheddar cheese

DIRECTIONS

1. In a saucepan melt butter, add onion, garlic and sauté until soft

2. Pour in heavy cream, chicken broth, stir in broccoli

3. Cover and continue cooking for 12-15 minutes

4. Add cheese and cook until melted

5. Stir in hot sauce and enjoy

KETO QUESO SOUP

Serves: 4
Prep Time: 10 Minutes
Cook Time: 30 Minutes
Total Time: 40 Minutes

INGREDIENTS

- 1 lb. chicken breast
- 1 tablespoon taco seasoning
- 1 tablespoon avocado oil
- 1 can diced green chilies
- 6-ounces cream cheese
- ½ cup heavy cream
- salt
- 2 cups chicken broth

DIRECTIONS

1. In an iron Dutch oven heat oil over medium heat stir in taco seasoning and cook for 1-2 minutes

2. Add broth, chicken and simmer for 20 minutes, remove chicken and shred

3. Stir in cream cheese and heavy cream into the soup, once the cheese has melted, add the chicken back to the soup, season with salt and serve

KETO CRAB SOUP

Serves: 6
Prep Time: 10   Minutes
Cook Time: 10   Minutes
Total Time: 20   Minutes

INGREDIENTS

- 1 tablespoon butter
- 1 tablespoon seasoning
- 6-ounces cream cheese
- ¾ cup parmesan cheese
- 1 lb. lump crabmeat

DIRECTIONS

1. In a pot melt butter and add seasoning, cream cheese and whisk until smooth

2. Add parmesan cheese, crab meat and reduce heat

3. Simmer until is done

4. Remove and serve

(SALAD)

KETO SALAD

Serves: 2
Prep Time: 10 Minutes
Cook Time: 10 Minutes
Total Time: 20 Minutes

INGREDIENTS

- 1 slice bacon
- 3-ounces chicken breast
- 1-ounce cheddar cheese
- 1 tablespoon olive oil
- 1 tablespoon apple cider vinegar
- ½ avocado
- 1 head romaine lettuce

DIRECTIONS

1. Chop all ingredients and place them in a bowl

2. Mix well and add pepper, oil and vinegar

KETO BROCCOLI SALAD

Serves: 2
Prep Time: 10   Minutes
Cook Time: 10   Minutes
Total Time: 20   Minutes

INGREDIENTS

- 20-ounce raw broccoli
- 1 cup bacon
- ½ red onion
- 1 cup avocado mayo
- 1 cup macadamia nuts
- ½ cup Monkfruit sweetener
- 1 tablespoon organic apple cider vinegar

DIRECTIONS

1. Place Macadamia Nuts in a blender and blend until smooth

2. Place all ingredients in a bowl and mix well, pour over Macadamia Nuts mixture and serve

KETO GREEN SPRING SALAD

Serves: 4
Prep Time: 10 Minutes
Cook Time: 30 Minutes
Total Time: 40 Minutes

INGREDIENTS

- 2-ounces mixed greens
- 2 tablespoons pine nuts
- 1 tablespoon raspberry vinaigrette
- 1 tablespoon parmesan
- 1 slice bacon
- salt and pepper

DIRECTIONS

1. Cook bacon until crispy

2. Place greens in a bowl with the rest of ingredients

3. Top with bacon and serve

KETO EGG SALAD

Serves: 4
Prep Time: 10 Minutes
Cook Time: 30 Minutes
Total Time: 40 Minutes

INGREDIENTS

- 6 eggs
- 2 celery stalks
- 2 green onion stalks
- 1 green pepper
- 1 tsp mustard
- 2/3 cup mayonnaise

DIRECTIONS

1. Hard boil eggs and remove to a bowl

2. Chop green pepper, onions and celery

3. In a bowl mix all the ingredients and serve

KETO CAESAR SALAD

Serves: 4
Prep Time: 10   Minutes
Cook Time: 30   Minutes
Total Time: 40   Minutes

INGREDIENTS

- 10 oz. chicken breasts
- 1 tablespoon olive oil
- salt
- 2 oz. bacon
- 6 oz. romaine lettuce
- 1 oz. parmesan cheese

DRESSING

- ½ cup mayonnaise
- 1 tablespoon chopped filets of anchovies
- 1 garlic clove
- 1 tablespoon mustard
- ½ lemon zest
- 1 tablespoon parmesan cheese

DIRECTIONS

1. In a bowl mix all ingredients for the dressing and set aside
2. Preheat oven to 400 F and place chicken breast in a baking dish and bake for 15-20 minutes
3. In a bowl place sliced chicken, all the salad ingredients, dressing and mix well

4. Serve with parmesan cheese

KETO PEPPERONI SALAD

Serves:4
Prep Time: 10 Minutes
Cook Time: 30 Minutes
Total Time: 40 Minutes

INGREDIENTS

- ½ avocado
- 12 slices pepperoni
- 1 oz. Mozzarella pears
- Italian seasoning

DIRECTIONS

1. In a bowl mix all ingredients and serve

KETO CHICKEN SALAD

Serves: 4
Prep Time: 10   Minutes
Cook Time: 30   Minutes
Total Time: 40   Minutes

INGREDIENTS

- 2 ribs celery
- ½ tsp pink Himalayan
- 1 tsp fresh dill
- ½ cup pecans
- 1 lb. chicken breast
- ½ cup mayo
- 1 tsp mustard

DIRECTIONS

1. Preheat oven to 425 F and bake chicken breast for 15-20 minutes

2. Remove chicken and cut into small pieces

3. In a bowl mix all ingredients and toss until chicken is fully coated

4. When ready, add dill and serve

KETO TUNA SALAD

Serves: 4
Prep Time: 10 Minutes
Cook Time: 30 Minutes
Total Time: 40 Minutes

INGREDIENTS

- 1 can tuna
- ½ tsp dill
- 1 boiled eg
- 1 slice bacon
- 1 tablespoon mayo
- 1 tablespoon sour cream
- 1 tsp mustard
- 1 tablespoon onion

DIRECTIONS

1. Prepare bacon, onion and boil egg

2. In a bowl place tuna, add egg and onion and the rest of ingredients

2. Top with bacon and serve

SPINACH SALAD

Serves: 4
Prep Time: 10   Minutes
Cook Time: 30   Minutes
Total Time: 40   Minutes

INGREDIENTS

- 2 cups spinach
- ½ avocado
- 1 strawberry

DRESSING

- 2 slices bacon
- 1 tablespoon avocado oil
- pinch red pepper flakes
- 1 tsp oregano
- ½ tsp garlic powder
- ½ tsp salt
- half lemon

DIRECTIONS

1. In a bowl mix all dressing ingredients

2. In another bowl mix salad ingredients and pour dressing over

3. Mix well and serve

KETO POTOTO SALAD

Serves: 1
Prep Time: 10   Minutes
Cook Time: 10   Minutes
Total Time: 20   Minutes

INGREDIENTS

- 1 cauliflower
- 1 tablespoon mustard
- 1 tsp celery seeds
- ½ tsp salt
- ½ cup celery
- 1 tsp dill
- ½ cup sour cream
- ½ cup mayonnaise
- 2 stalks green onions
- 2 hard boiled eggs
- 1 tablespoon white vinegar

DIRECTIONS

1. In a bowl prepare dressing by whisking together sour cream, celery seed, salt, mayonnaise, vinegar and mustard

2. In another bowl mix salad ingredient, pour dressing and mix well

DINNER RECIPES

KETO MONGOLAIN BEEF

Serves:2
Prep Time: 10   Minutes
Cook Time: 10   Minutes
Total Time: 20   Minutes

INGREDIENTS

- 1 lb. flat iron steak
- ½ cup coconut oil
- 2 green onions

LOW CARB MONGOLIAN BEEF MARINADE

- ½ cup coconut aminos
- 1 tsp ginger
- 1 clove garlic

DIRECTIONS

1. Cut the flat iron steak into thin slices

2. Add the beef to a ziplock bag and add coconut aminos, garlic and ginger, marinate for 1 hour

3. Add coconut oil to a wok and cook beef on high heat for 2-3 minutes

4. Add green onions, cook for another 1-2 minutes

5. Remove and serve

PEPPERONI KETO PIZZA

Serves: 2
Prep Time: 10   Minutes
Cook Time: 10   Minutes
Total Time: 20   Minutes

INGREDIENTS

- 1 cauli'flour foods crust
- 2 oz. pepperoni
- ½ cup pizza sauce
- salt
- 2-ounces fresh mozzarella
- ½ cup jalapeno

DIRECTIONS

1. Preheat oven to 375 F and place pizza crust on a vented pizza pan, cook for 8-10 minutes

2. Add mozzarella, sauce, pepperoni and jalapeno

3. Place back in the oven for 5-6 minutes

4. Remove and serve

QUICK KETO PIZZA

Serves: 4
Prep Time: 10   Minutes
Cook Time: 10   Minutes
Total Time: 10   Minutes

INGREDIENTS

PIZZA CRUST

- 2 eggs
- 1 tablespoon parmesan cheese
- 1 tablespoon husk powder
- ½ tsp Italian seasoning
- salt
- 2 tsp frying oil

TOPPINGS

- 1 oz. mozzarella cheese
- 2 tablespoons. Tomato sauce
- 1 tablespoon chopped basil

DIRECTIONS

1. In a bowl mix all pizza crust ingredients

2. Spoon the mixture into a pan, cook for 1 minute per side

3. Add cheese, tomato sauce and broil for 1-2 minutes until cheese is bubbling

MUSHROOMS PIZZA

Serves: 2
Prep Time: 10 Minutes
Cook Time: 15 Minutes
Total Time: 25 Minutes

INGREDIENTS

- ¼ cup rao's marinara
- pepperoni
- sliced baby bella mushrooms
- sliced ripe olives
- mozzarella

DIRECTIONS

1. Preheat oven to 375 F

2. Spray a pie plate with a non-stick cooking spray

3. Spread marinara on bottom of pie plate

4. Layer mushrooms, pepperoni, olives and top with mozzarella

5. Bake for 10 minutes and serve

BUFFALO KETO CHICKEN TENDERS

Serves: 2
Prep Time: 10   Minutes
Cook Time: 30   Minutes
Total Time: 40   Minutes

INGREDIENTS

- 1 lb. chicken breast tenders
- 1 cup almond flour
- 1 egg
- 1 tablespoon heavy whipping cream
- 5 oz. buffalo sauce
- salt

DIRECTIONS

1. Preheat oven to 325 F

2. Season chicken with salt, pepper and almond flour

3. Beat 1 egg with heavy cream

4. Dip each tender in the egg and then into seasoned almond flour

5. Place tenders on a baking sheet and bake for 25 minutes or until crispy

6. Remove and serve

KETO LASAGNA

Serves: 4
Prep Time: 10   Minutes
Cook Time: 30   Minutes
Total Time: 40   Minutes

INGREDIENTS

- 1 lb. ground beef
- 1 cup sauce
- ¾ cup mozzarella
- 6 tablespoons ricotta
- salt, onion powder, Italian seasoning

DIRECTIONS

1. Preheat oven to 350 F, brown beef and season

2. Being to layer a deep dish with noodle, ricotta, sauce mix and sprinkle with mozzarella, top with cheese

3. Bake for 20-25 minutes

4. Remove and serve

KETO PARMESAN CASSEROLE

Serves: 3
Prep Time: 10   Minutes
Cook Time: 30   Minutes
Total Time: 40   Minutes

INGREDIENTS

- 2 cups cooked chicken
- ½ tsp basil
- 1 slice bacon
- ½ cup marinara sauce
- ½ tsp red pepper flakes
- ¾ cup mozzarella cheese
- ½ cup Parmesan cheese

DIRECTIONS

1. Preheat the oven to 325 F

2. Lay out the chicken in the pan and spread the marinara sauce all over

3. Dredge the top with parmesan, red pepper flakes, mozzarella and sprinkle bacon and basil

4. Bake for 20-25 minutes, remove and serve

KETO CHEESE MEATBALLS

Serves: 2
Prep Time: 10 Minutes
Cook Time: 10 Minutes
Total Time: 20 Minutes

INGREDIENTS

- ½ lbs. beef mince
- 2 tablespoons parmesan cheese
- ½ tsp salt
- ½ tsp pepper
- ¼ lbs. cheese
- 1 tsp garlic powder

DIRECTIONS

1. Cut the cheese into cubes

2. Mix all dry ingredients with the ground beef

3. Wrap the cubes of cheese in mince and pan fry the meatballs

KETO CHEESY BACON CHICKEN

Serves: 4
Prep Time: 10   Minutes
Cook Time: 30   Minutes
Total Time: 40   Minutes

INGREDIENTS

- 5 chicken breasts
- 2 tablespoons seasoning rub
- ½ lbs. bacon
- 3 oz. shredded cheddar
- barbecue sauce

DIRECTIONS

1. Preheat oven to 375 F and spray a baking sheet with cooking spray

2. Rub both sides of chicken breast with seasoning rub and top with bacon, bake for 25 minutes

3. Remove from oven, sprinkle with cheese and serve

KETO CHEESEBURGER

Serves: 2
Prep Time: 10   Minutes
Cook Time: 60   Minutes
Total Time: 70   Minutes

INGREDIENTS

- 2 lbs. ground beef
- 2 eggs
- ½ cup grated parmesan
- 1 small onion
- 1 tsp salt
- 1 tsp garlic powder
- ½ cup cheddar cheese

DIRECTIONS

1. In a bowl mix all ingredients except cheddar cheese, add the end add cheese cubes

2. Place mixture into a sprayed oven dish and form a meatloaf shape

3. Bake at 325 F for 50 minutes

4. Remove and serve

DESSERT RECIPES

(CAKE)

CHEESECAKE KETO FAT BOMBS

Serves: 12
Prep Time: 10   Minutes
Cook Time: 10   Minutes
Total Time: 20   Minutes

INGREDIENTS

- 5 oz. cream cheese
- 2 oz. frozen strawberries
- 2 oz. butter
- 1 oz. swerve sweetener
- 1 tsp vanilla extract

DIRECTIONS

1. Puree the strawberries using a blender

2. In a bowl mix sweetener, vanilla, pureed strawberries and mix well

3. Microwave cream cheese and combine with the rest of ingredients

4. Add butter to the mixture and mix with an electric mixer

5. Divide into 10-12 round silicone molds and freeze for 1-2 hours before serving

KETO BROWNIES

Serves: 12
Prep Time: 10 Minutes
Cook Time: 20 Minutes
Total Time: 30 Minutes

INGREDIENTS

- ½ cup almond flour
- ½ tsp baking powder
- 1 tablespoon instant coffee
- 2 oz. chocolate
- 1 egg
- ½ tsp vanilla extract
- ½ cup cacao powder
- 2/3 cup Erythritol
- 8 tablespoons utter

DIRECTIONS

1. Preheat oven to 325 F

2. In a medium bowl whisk almond flour, baking powder, Erythritol, cocoa powder and instant coffee

3. In another bowl melt chocolate and butter and whisk in the eggs and vanilla

4. Add to dry ingredients and mix well

5. Transfer batter into baking dish and bake for 20 minutes

6. Remove and serve

KETO ICE CREAM

Serves: 2
Prep Time: 10   Minutes
Cook Time: 20   Minutes
Total Time: 30   Minutes

INGREDIENTS

- 2 cups heavy cream
- 1 tablespoon milk powder
- ½ tsp xanthum gum
- 1 tsp vanilla extract
- 1 cup whole milk
- ½ cup truvia baking blend

DIRECTIONS

1. In a bowl mix milk powder, sweetener, xanthum gum

2. Pour in cream, vanilla extract, milk and mix until sweetener is dissolved

3. Pour into ice cream maker and churn until set

4. Serve when ready

KETO EGG CREPES

Serves: 2
Prep Time: 10 Minutes
Cook Time: 10 Minutes
Total Time: 20 Minutes

INGREDIENTS

- 5 eggs
- 5 oz. cream cheese
- 1 tsp cinnamon
- 1 tablespoon sugar substitute
- butter

FILLING

- 7 tablespoons butter
- ½ cup sugar substitute
- 1 tablespoon cinnamon

DIRECTIONS

1. Blend all of the crepe ingredients until smooth

2. Pour batter into the pan and cook 1-2 minutes per side

3. Remove and pour mixture over the crepes

4. For crepes mixture mix cinnamon and sweetener in a bowl

5. Serve when ready

KETO NAAN

Serves:4
Prep Time: 10   Minutes
Cook Time: 30   Minutes
Total Time: 40   Minutes

INGREDIENTS

- ½ cup coconut flour
- 1 tablespoon psyllium husk
- 1 tablespoon ghee
- ½ tsp baking powder
- ½ tsp salt
- 1 cup boiling water

DIRECTIONS

1. In a bowl mix all ingredients and refrigerate

2. Divine the dough into 6 balls

3. Heat a cast iron skillet over medium heat and place ice naan ball

4. Cook for 2-3 minutes remove and serve

PEANUT BUTTER COOKIES

Serves: 12
Prep Time: 10   Minutes
Cook Time: 30   Minutes
Total Time: 40   Minutes

INGREDIENTS

- 1 cup peanut butter
- 1 tsp vanilla
- 1 tsp baking powder
- ½ tsp salt
- ½ cup keto sweetener
- 1 egg

DIRECTIONS

1. Preheat oven to 325 F

2. Cream together all ingredients

3. Refrigerate for 15-20 minutes

4. Roll dough into balls and place on a parchment paper

5. Bake for 12-15 minutes

BUTTERY KETO CREPES

Serves: 2
Prep Time: 10 Minutes
Cook Time: 10 Minutes
Total Time: 20 Minutes

INGREDIENTS

- 3 eggs
- ½ tsp vanilla extract
- ½ tsp cinnamon
- 3 oz. cream cheese
- 2 tsp sweetener
- 2 tablespoons butter

DIRECTIONS

1. In a blender place all the ingredients and blend until smooth

2. In a skillet pour batter and cook each crepe for 1-2 minutes per side or until ready

3. Remove and serve with berries, maple syrup or jam

KETO LEMON FAT BOMB

Serves:4
Prep Time: 10 Minutes
Cook Time: 10 Minutes
Total Time: 20 Minutes

INGREDIENTS

- ½ cup coconut oil
- 3 tablespoons butter
- 3 oz. cream cheese
- 2 tsp lemon juice
- 2 tsp sugar substitute

DIRECTIONS

1. Place all ingredients in a mixing bowl and mix thoroughly

2. Spoon 2 tablespoons into cupcake holders and freeze

3. Remove and serve

PEANUT BUTTER BALLS

Serves: 4
Prep Time: 10   Minutes
Cook Time: 30   Minutes
Total Time: 40   Minutes

INGREDIENTS

- 1 cup peanuts finely chopped
- 1 cup peanut butter
- 1 cup powdered sweetener
- 6 oz. sugar free chocolate chips

DIRECTIONS

1. In a bowl mix peanut butter, sweetener, chopped peanuts, divide dough into 12 pieces and shape into balls and place on a wax paper

2. Melt chocolate and dip each peanut butter ball in the chocolate and place back on the wax paper

3. Refrigerate and serve

NUT FREE KETO BROWNIE

Serves: 8
Prep Time: 10   Minutes
Cook Time: 20   Minutes
Total Time: 30   Minutes

INGREDIENTS

- 5 eggs
- ¼ lb. butter
- 2 oz. cocoa
- ½ tsp baking powder
- 2 tsp vanilla
- ¼ lb. cream cheese
- 3 tablespoons sweetener of choice

DIRECTIONS

1. Place all the ingredients in a lender and blend until smooth

2. Pour mixture into a baking dish

3. Bake at 325 F for 20 minutes

4. Remove slice into squares and serve

SMOOTHIES

COFFEE SMOOTHIE

Serves:1
Prep Time: 5   Minutes
Cook Time: 5   Minutes
Total Time: 10   Minutes

INGREDIENTS

- 5 oz. cold coffee
- 3 oz. heavy cream
- 3 oz. almond milk
- 1 oz. sugar free chocolate syrup
- 1 oz. caramel syrup
- 1 tablespoon cocoa
- 12 oz. ice

DIRECTIONS

1. In a blender place all the ingredients and blend until smooth

2. Pour in a glass and serve

CHAI PUMPKIN SMOOTHIE

Serves: 1
Prep Time: 5   Minutes
Cook Time: 5   Minutes
Total Time: 10   Minutes

INGREDIENTS

- ¾ cup coconut milk
- 2 tablespoon pumpkin puree
- 1 tablespoon MCT oil
- 1 tsp chai tea
- 1 tsp alcohol free vanilla
- ½ tsp pumpkin pie spice
- ½ frozen avocado

DIRECTIONS

1. In a blender place all the ingredients and blend until smooth

2. Pour in a glass and serve

CASHEW SMOOTHIE

Serves:1
Prep Time: 5   Minutes
Cook Time: 5   Minutes
Total Time: 10 Minutes

INGREDIENTS

- 1 cup cashew mik
- 1 tablespoon keto MCT oil
- 1 tablespoon keto nut butter
- 1 tsp maca powder
- 1 handful ice

DIRECTIONS

1. In a blender place all the ingredients and blend until smooth

2. Pour in a glass and serve

BREAKFAST SMOOTHIE

Serves:1
Prep Time: 5   Minutes
Cook Time: 5   Minutes
Total Time: 10   Minutes

INGREDIENTS

- ½ cup almond milk
- ½ cup coconut milk
- ½ coconut yoghurt
- ½ tsp stevia
- 3 strawberries

DIRECTIONS

1.   In a blender place all the ingredients and blend until smooth

2.   Pour in a glass and serve

KETO MILKSHAKE SMOOTHIE

Serves: 1
Prep Time: 5   Minutes
Cook Time: 5   Minutes
Total Time: 10 Minutes

INGREDIENTS

- 6 oz. plain almond milk
- 3 oz. crushed ice
- 1 oz. heavy whipping cream
- 1 oz. raspberries
- ¾ oz. sweetener of choice
- ½ oz. cream cheese

DIRECTIONS

1. In a blender place all the ingredients and blend until smooth

2. Pour in a glass and serve

AVOCADO SMOOTHIE

Serves: 1
Prep Time: 5   Minutes
Cook Time: 5   Minutes
Total Time: 10   Minutes

INGREDIENTS

- ½ avocado
- 2 tablespoons cocoa powder
- 2/3 cup coconut milk
- ½ cup crushed ice
- ½ cup water
- pinch of salt
- 1 tsp lime juice
- stevia

DIRECTIONS

1. In a blender place all the ingredients and blend until smooth

2. Pour in a glass and serve

COLLAGEN SMOOTHIE

Serves: 1
Prep Time: 5   Minutes
Cook Time: 5   Minutes
Total Time: 10   Minutes

INGREDIENTS

- 4 ice cubes
- ½ avocado
- 1 scoop keto chocolate collagen
- 1 tablespoon chia seeds
- 1 tablespoon almond butter
- ¾ cup heavy whipping cream
- 1 cup water

DIRECTIONS

1. In a blender place all the ingredients and blend until smooth

2. Pour in a glass and serve

FAT BOMB SMOOTHIE

Serves: 1
Prep Time: 5   Minutes
Cook Time: 5   Minutes
Total Time: 10   Minutes

INGREDIENTS

- 2.5 oz avocado
- 1 scoop collagen
- 1 tablespoon cacao powder
- 1 cup almond milk
- 1 cup ice

DIRECTIONS

1. In a blender place all the ingredients and blend until smooth

2. Pour in a glass and serve

CINNAMON SMOOTHIE

Serves: 1
Prep Time: 5   Minutes
Cook Time: 5   Minutes
Total Time: 10   Minutes

INGREDIENTS

- ½ cup coconut milk
- ½ cup water
- 2 ice cubes
- 1 tablespoon coconut oil
- ½ tsp cinnamon
- 1 tablespoon chia seeds
- ½ cup vanilla protein powder

DIRECTIONS

1. In a blender place all the ingredients and blend until smooth

2. Pour in a glass and serve

TROPICAL SMOOTHIE

Serves: 1
Prep Time: 5   Minutes
Cook Time: 5   Minutes
Total Time: 10   Minutes

INGREDIENTS

- ½ tsp banana extract
- ½ tsp blueberry extract
- ½ tsp mango extract
- stevia
- 1 tablespoon oil
- ½ cup sour cream
- ice cubes
- ¾ cup coconut milk

DIRECTIONS

1. In a blender place all the ingredients and blend until smooth

2. Pour in a glass and serve

Conclusion

And here we are at the conclusion!

Now you have reached the end of the book 16.8 DIET and the beginning of a new life in which you will be master of your body. Everything you read in the book is to help you love yourself, be happy and lose weight naturally, and so it will be. It doesn't matter if you believe what you have read or not, you just have to follow all the instructions. I think I told you everything you need to get back in shape and finally lose all that excess fat and maybe even get a screaming abdomen out!

This book contains the best strategies to help you lose weight. If you follow my advice I assure you that you will get excellent results, but remember that you will get them only if you put effort and perseverance. If you have read the book in one breath, now you have to decide whether to be a lazy woman who does not act despite having golden strategies in your hand, or you can get busy and get results. If you have decided to get busy, then start reading and studying the book from the beginning and turn what you read into ACTION! You can lose weight, but this is up to you, it is up to you to do the simple daily actions that will make your body thin through the new habits you will learn, and certain habits are made to last a lifetime.

So, don't wait, get busy today!

Read - Understand - Apply - Persevere - Reach the goal!

I wish you to achieve your goal of losing weight and living a happy and joyful life.

Your friend **Lisa Campbell**

***

P.S. Before I leave you I want to thank you for reading my book! If you liked it, then could you please take a minute to write an honest (hopefully positive) review on Amazon.com or Audible.com? I would appreciate it very much, as it will help me to read this book to more people!

Thanks, thanks, thanks.

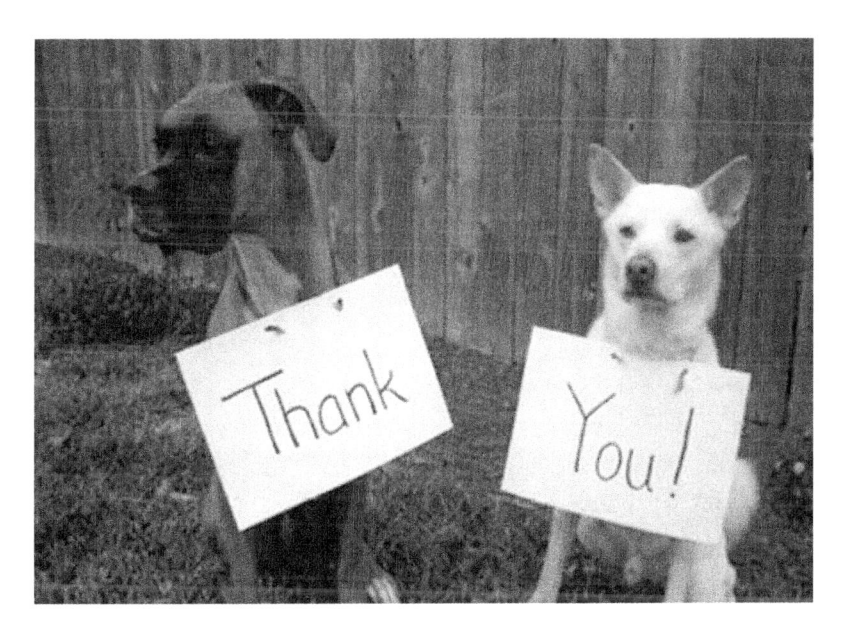

***

Thor & Luna, MY DOGS ... ☺

Printed in Great Britain
by Amazon